THAT WAS NOT A MUSCLE

How Counterstrain is Transforming My Pain Therapy Practice

COACH IZZY

For permission requests, write to the publisher at:

Mar en Hoguera Media, LLC
9431 Coppertop Loop NE
Suite 102 A1 – A2
Bainbridge Island, WA 98110

First Edition, June 2026.

ISBN: 978-0-98356-614-4

That Was not A Muscle – How Counterstrain is Transforming my Pain Therapy Practice
by Israel A. Sanchez AKA Coach Izzy

Models: Timary Daniel, Erica St. Clair, Izzy Sanchez
IIS Hypothesis Flowchart reproduced with permission of Brian Tuckey.

Printed in the United States of America
Library of Congress Cataloging-in-Publication Data:

[To be obtained]

To CP, my wife, my love.
Your love and sacrifice made
all of this possible.

To my family, for the courage
to heal together and be stronger
than ever.

TABLE OF CONTENTS

MEDICAL DISCLAIMER

The information presented in this book is intended for educational and informational purposes only. It is not intended as a substitute for professional medical advice, diagnosis, or treatment. The scientific explanations and procedural descriptions of Strain-Counterstrain, Fascial Counterstrain, and/or Counterstrain provided herein are based on current understanding and research but may not reflect all perspectives in the medical or therapeutic communities.

Readers are advised to consult a licensed healthcare provider before beginning any treatment, including Strain-Counterstrain, Fascial Counterstrain, and/or Counterstrain, especially if they have preexisting medical conditions or concerns. The authors and publishers of this book are not responsible for any adverse effects or consequences resulting from the use of any suggestions, procedures, or exercises described in this text.

The content of this book is not intended to establish a standard of care or to replace the expertise and judgment of qualified healthcare professionals. Always seek the advice of your physician or other qualified health provider with any questions you may have regarding a medical condition or treatment.

Use of the techniques and information contained in this book is at the reader's own risk.

COOKING NOODLES

David D. looked at Tim Hodges with a squint, mouth agape.

"Say that again?" David asked.

The witty Alaskan physical therapist who made the trek to Oregon every other Friday to take part in the Counterstrain Mastery Program, now the Counterstrain Academy, was notorious for peppering his statements with colorful analogies.

Tim smiled. "You can determine whether the tender points are anterior or posterior by testing the location on the cranial scan."

David leaned forward. "For real?"

Tim nodded, reveling in delivering mind-blowing information.

"Tim, man, you just cooked my noodle!" David said, letting his words flow with the emotions of profound revelations, summarizing what all of us felt.

This took place in the winter of 2014 and the excitement is as vivid today as it was then. My heart fills with gratitude whenever I recall the amazement I experienced the first time I met Tim Hodges LMT, JSCCI, CACI, CSC III, in the fall of 2011, a day that reshaped the course of my career as a pain therapist. Little did I know I'd be immersing in the astonishing world of Counterstrain during one of the most exciting evolutionary periods of its history.

This indirect, powerful, gentle, and effective modality became my primary discipline when it started producing results where other modalities fell short. I credit Counterstrain with skyrocketing my success rate and saving my time and sanity.

But my attachment to Counterstrain goes beyond the therapy room. Counterstrain allowed me to help my family in ways I could've never imagined. From helping my wife when her back pain seemed hopeless, to cementing the bonds between me and my Dad as I helped him with his pains—an experience that I'll forever treasure now that he's no longer with us.

It is my objective to present the theoretical rationale of this magnificent modality and its human aspect. And it is my objective to do so without getting you lost in the rich physiological layers that the aspiring Counterstrain therapist must master to become competent and effective. My illustrations also reflect this goal, which meant sacrificing detailed textbook accuracy in exchange for conveying the general concept. I want to simplify this journey but without falling into the trap of oversimplification. The way I see it, *oversimplification is misinformation disguised as user-friendly knowledge.* Ultimately, though, Counterstrain is a modality that must be experienced to be fully understood, and we can start by getting acquainted with its principles.

One of my concerns was that the information I'm about to share would be exploited by hucksters and copycats but as the system evolved, I realized that even if someone secretly recorded the techniques, they wouldn't be able to use them—and even if they did, they'd be more likely to cause adverse reactions than to bring relief. That is because *Counterstrain is not about techniques but about the undeniable physiological principles dictating the application of those techniques.* It would be like a non-dancer trying to imitate an experienced dancer. The moves may be copied but not the flavor or flow because they come from the embodiment of musical and rhythmic principles—something the non-dancer lacks. Similarly, the success of the Counterstrain therapist lies in the embodiment and application of the physiological principles governing our modality, not necessarily in the techniques. While the techniques get constantly refined and changed, the principles remain untouched.

I look forward to sharing my journey with you.

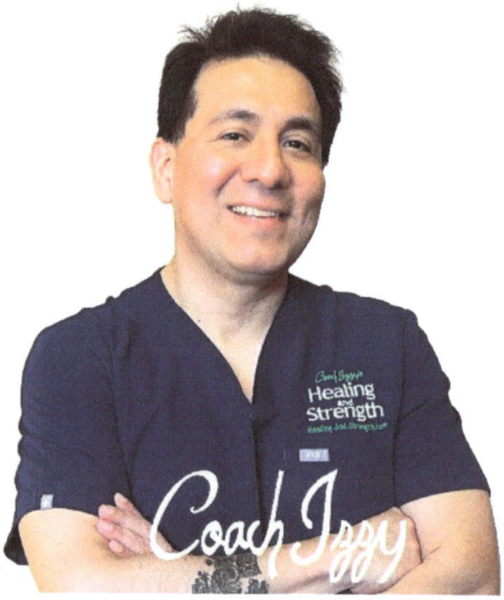

HOW THIS BOOK IS ORGANIZED

I started this book in late 2013, at a time when it seemed that Fascial Counterstrain (FCS) was approaching its completion as a therapeutic system that could be reliably segmented for instruction.

But the system was not anywhere close to completion—and it still is not. The ever-increasing complexity of the cases arriving at our practices showed us we still had ways to go and much to learn. Advances in medical research, advances in our assessment methodology, the advent of the Counterstrain Convention, and the publication of the Counterstrain rationale in a scientific journal in 2021, and then of the methodology in another scientific journal in 2025, meant multiple rewrites. For a while, I contemplated ditching this project.

But our clients, medical providers, and potential therapists kept asking. They wanted to know what made Counterstrain so effective and how we ended up adopting a modality whose principles defy established norms. Whenever they asked, I'd present the physiological principles in a user-friendly format and provided scientific resources when needed.

The reward was seeing their eyes light up as the modality that made such a difference in their lives began to make sense. This gave me the energy and direction to put it all together. I share the governing physiological principles and applications, but I also share the human aspects of Counterstrain. Based on the aforementioned, the book is organized in the following segments:

- **Beginnings and Differences.** Who discovered Counterstrain and how? In this segment I explain how the system came to be and the differences between the original system and its evolved format. I also address common questions to help eliminate the confusion that's still rampant when trying to compare them.

- **The Vicious Cycle in Pain Therapy.** Never did I contemplate a career in manual therapy medicine until life opened my eyes to the frustrating vicious cycle in pain therapy and showed me how others shared the same frustrations. But there's hope in breaking the cycle.

- **From the Training Floor to the Treatment Table.** Driven by my mission, life would stealthily guide me from strength and conditioning to manual therapy medicine through events and lessons, some elating and some painful, ultimately giving me a new professional direction.

- **That Was Not a Muscle.** The frustrations from the increasingly complex cases arriving to my practice made it clear that I was overlooking an important component. A crucial encounter would forever reshape the course of my career and put me in the most demanding but satisfying path in manual therapy medicine.
- **The Nuts and Bolts of Fascial Counterstrain.** The technical segment of this book, in which you'll get an overview of the physiological principles, structures, and interactions involved in what creates the experience we call pain and what perpetuates it. You will learn how a common element of the healing process could be responsible and how FCS addresses it.
- **The Counterstrain Experience.** There a couple of misconceptions that interfere with the understanding of Counterstrain. One can be addressed directly but the other is more abstract and prevalent, and needs to be seen from a different lens. You will also become acquainted with some of the factors the proficient therapist must consider to deliver effective treatment.
- **Counterstrain and You.** This is your guide in how to approach Counterstrain when you're ready to incorporate it in your life as a client or as a therapist. We'll go over some of the most common areas of confusion, and how you can maximize your session benefits. In addition, those who wish to pursue Counterstrain as a career will find some handy guides and resources.

The one thing you won't find is technique descriptions or demonstrations. There will be pictures showing general approaches but unless you're a practitioner, you won't know what's going on. This is done intentionally for two reasons.

One, the current techniques are the intellectual property of Brian Tuckey PT, JSCCI, OCS, CSC III, the originator of Fascial Counterstrain. He greenlights demonstrations when appropriate, and this is not one of those circumstances. Two, applying the techniques without embodying their governing principles makes one, at best, ineffective. At worst, it makes one an incompetent liability that could provoke undesired effects on unsuspecting clients.

For those eager to truly understand Counterstrain, you can explore the citations and resources in this book. However, nothing beats getting involved in the field as a client or as a therapist to fully grasp the immensity of Counterstrain.

BEGINNINGS AND DIFFERENCES

STRAIN-COUNTERSTRAIN OR FASCIAL COUNTERSTRAIN?

The Only Consistency in Life is Inevitable Change.

Which is it? Why the different denominations? Aren't they the same technique after all? The answer depends on whom you ask, and what I'm about to tell you is based on my exposure to the system during a key evolutionary period.

If you heard of, or received, the modality prior to 2015, chances are that you know it as *Strain-Counterstrain (SCS)*. Those who experienced it in the latter years probably know it as *Fascial Counterstrain (FCS)*. While this may seem an issue of semantics, the reality is much deeper as Strain-Counterstrain and Fascial Counterstrain encompass two entities that share similar principles but differ in rationale and approach. Yet they're also an unbreakable continuum and it's undeniable that the latter could not have existed without the creation of the former. To better understand them, it's important to recognize their origins.

One ponders about the brilliant mind that had the insight to tap into this neglected component of our physiology and turn it into a therapeutic modality. Perhaps a sage poring over obscure books and research papers, conducting experiments in neurology and physiology, until arriving at the governing principles of the modality.

But those of us immersed in the field know that the late Dr. Lawrence Jones, DO—the insightful healer who developed the foundations of the system in 1955—never shied away from sharing the true origins. Like many of the discoveries that shaped history and changed the world, Dr. Jones stumbled upon his system by accident.

Strain-Counterstrain (SCS)

Dr. Jones tells us of the case of a thirty-year-old patient who, despite being treated by other doctors, had been dealing with debilitating back pain for nearly six months [1] [2]. Dr. Jones admits that he was also about to concede failure after six weeks of unsuccessful treatment. That's when the patient suggested that he might respond better if he could find a comfortable position to sleep since the pain regularly disrupted his slumber.

Dr. Jones agreed and proceeded to stretch and contract the patient in different directions, using the patient's feedback until finding the position that felt best. Dr. Jones was puzzled at what he called "the wild and grotesque position" that resulted from all the adjustments, but that was the most comfortable the patient had been in a long time, so Dr. Jones just propped him with some pillows and a chair while he treated another patient.

Dr. Jones returned after about twenty minutes and found that the patient had been so relaxed he had dozed off. When Dr. Jones woke him up and helped him up, the patient was thrilled at how much better he was feeling. So much so that he was finally able to stand upright after all those months of pain and restriction.

That was the spark the brilliant and intuitive Dr. Jones needed to investigate the possible mechanisms of the phenomenon and develop his work [2]. He theorized that the sustained position unloaded aberrant protective reflex arcs—a nervous system reset, if you will. He initially called his system *Spontaneous Release by Positioning*, then *Strain and Counterstrain* and eventually *Strain-Counterstrain*, a therapeutic modality that follows a core principle:

Follow the direction of ease.

Dr. Jones had noticed that many palpable restrictions and dysfunctions contracted in a specific direction and that they were accompanied by tender points—specific inflamed spots sensitive to touch—that would melt away when the segment was guided into its direction of ease. Treatment consisted of guiding the affected segment into this direction while using the tender points to monitor the effectiveness of the treatment.

Despite the virtual absence of relevant research, Dr. Jones continued evolving his system, creating about 200 different treatments. He eventually presented his findings in the article *Spontaneous Release by Positioning* in 1963. But in 1975 another researcher, Dr. Irvin Korr, showed interest in SCS and attributed the *aberrant reflex arcs* (meaning reflex arcs that should not be there) to the musculoskeletal proprioceptors [3]. While this rationale was satisfactory, it could not explain the exceptions that would not follow musculoskeletal patterns. It wasn't until the '90s when Dr. Richard

Van Buskirk theorized that dysregulated sensory neurons, or *nociceptors* (more on that later), could be at the core of the aberrant reflexes and the effects felt during treatment [4]. No other researchers conducted studies on SCS at that point.

It did not matter. Dr. Jones continued investigating, developing, refining his work, and training a select group of therapists who became his four original certified instructors. The Jones' Strain-Counterstrain method remained—with some exceptions—unchanged for the next five decades.

How is SCS applied?

I have a fondness for the Strain-Counterstrain approach, as it was my introduction to this brilliant healing modality. I immediately fell in love with its elegant gentleness. As a bonus, the skills I mastered through SCS allowed me to easily transition to some of the newer Fascial Counterstrain modules in which positional finesse, not soft tissue gliding, is required.

Before applying SCS techniques, the therapist will analyze the area of complaint and start looking for specific *tender points*, which in Counterstrain are evidence of dysfunction. The therapist may also analyze other anatomical segments if the complaint area lacks distinctive tender points. For instance, some hand, elbow, or shoulder pains are driven by dysfunctions in the ribs or spinal joints rather than the upper extremities. Once a specific tender point has been identified, the therapist will place the affected segment in a predetermined position for ninety seconds to two minutes, always going in its direction of ease and monitoring the tender point. When the time is concluded, the affected segment should be freer, less painful, and the tender point significantly reduced, if not gone. The therapist will continue this process for a specific amount of time, or until they feel the client has reached a satisfactory state.

This is how SCS was practiced for over five decades. The complete set of techniques was presented in four different modules—three of them addressing different regions of the body, and one that integrated and refined them all. Some students pursued this path to the fullest while others only added some of the techniques to their repertoires, but it was the more proficient practitioners who earned the reputation as the go-to people for unsolvable cases.

Then the inevitable happened. The cases increased in complexity to the point at which the once highly effective techniques barely made a difference.

It would've seemed that the method had met its limitations until one of Dr. Jones' four original instructors realized that the reach of his mentor's methodology was far more profound than what was established. His extensive background in different manual therapy modalities gave him the insight to apply the core SCS principles in a different fashion, thus tapping into physiological realms never considered in standard manual therapy medicine. The name of this instructor is **Brian Tuckey, PT, JSCCI, OCS, CSC III**, and he is the therapist responsible not only for the evolution of the system, but also for shattering the paradigms of manual therapy medicine, thus permanently reshaping its future.

Fascial Counterstrain (FCS)

If you ever stumbled upon Brian Tuckey, you would never know you did unless you personally knew him. You would never know that this pleasant, unassuming man with whom you probably shared a chat over coffee could be responsible for transforming not only the manual therapy medicine field but also the way in which we understand our bodies.

That's Brian, a man not comfortable with praise but quite at home solving the most complex pain and dysfunction cases, and sharing his developments with those seeking his guidance. Brian officially introduced his methodology in 2008 with the *Counterstrain for the Viscera and Lymphatic/ Venous Systems* course [5]. He's been unstoppable since then, thus creating techniques for veins, arteries, nerves in all their systemic divisions, meningeal layers, pericardial layers, visceral ligaments, spinal ligaments, tendons, cartilage, periosteum, adipose tissues, myofascia, and scar tissue.

When Brian is not introducing new modules, he's busy conducting extensive research to refine and optimize his existing work. A treatment that could've taken us half an hour three years before can be done in ten minutes or less, thanks to updates.

How is FCS Applied?

The application of FCS is so unorthodox that it throws off those who—in an effort to understand it—compare it to other modalities. While some aspects may seem familiar, most won't be, and the more one tries to compare them, the more confused one gets. Yes, Fascial Counterstrain is radically different, not just from Strain-Counterstrain but also from its own earlier versions. I'll go briefly over the process, but you'll get a lot more details in the **Nuts and Bolts of Fascial Counterstrain** chapter.

The success of the FCS therapist lies in their mastery of anatomy and physiology, as well as in their mastery of proprietary assessment techniques that necessitate specific palpatory skills. The FCS therapist will start by exploring the affected area and surrounding structures via joint motion and range of motion testing to identify the segment with the most restrictions and corresponding tender points. Next, the therapist must identify whether the restrictions and tender points are specific to the area or being driven by other segments. This is accomplished through a combination of motion testing, inhibitory techniques, and the most powerful tool in the Fascial Counterstrain assessment arsenal: *The Cranial Scan.*

We use the cranial scan to verify and refine our findings as well as the hierarchy and sequence of treatment. The cranial scan corroborates whether the restrictions and tenderness found in the affected area are the result of local protective mechanisms, or the result of protective mechanisms elsewhere.

Based on the findings, the therapist will direct their attention to a specific tender point and commence treatment via a soft-tissue glide, or body positioning, or a combination of both. If the assessment was accurate, the affected segment will start experiencing a positive change when moved in its direction of ease, and the glide or positioning should last between fifteen to forty-five seconds for most cases. After the allotted time, the tender point will be substantially reduced or gone, and the restricted segments will be freer.

The therapist will then repeat the process of combining motion testing, tender point identification, cranial scan, and treatment until time runs out or the client reaches stability.

It is important to clarify that we do *not* treat tender points. Instead, we *indirectly* treat their symptom-driving structures. I think of tender points as proxies since each tender point is an expression of a specific structure and those structures involve far more than the typical musculoskeletal culprits. Considering that the combined number of tender points representing the structures from all the currently treated physiological systems surpasses well over a thousand, it's easy to see why the combination of segment motion testing, inhibitory techniques, tender point identification, and cranial scan is crucial for efficient and effective treatment.

Which One is Better?

That is a question I often get from therapists who are trying to figure out the most efficient way to start their path in Counterstrain, or from clients who have received both versions and now have a harder time understanding the system. *Is one approach better than the other?*

The problem with this question is that it should not even be a question in the first place. One approach is the evolution of the other, thus, they have the duality of being similar but not comparable. Dr. Jones worked with the research, understanding, and technology that were current at his time and did incredible work with what he had.

The point of contention is that the fascial model addresses physiological systems that were not covered by the original SCS, and the effects and aftermath of FCS are significantly different from

SCS. While all of this is true, we must not forget that the fascial method would not exist if it hadn't been for Dr. Jones' work. Even Brian Tuckey himself has said so repeatedly.

I'm convinced that it's beneficial for practitioners to be familiar with both approaches, as there will be instances in which the SCS approach will be preferable. For instance, Counterstrain guidelines advise against fascial glides of the fascial structures located by the front of the neck in certain populations. That's when treating by specifically positioning the head and neck via SCS will accomplish the goal.

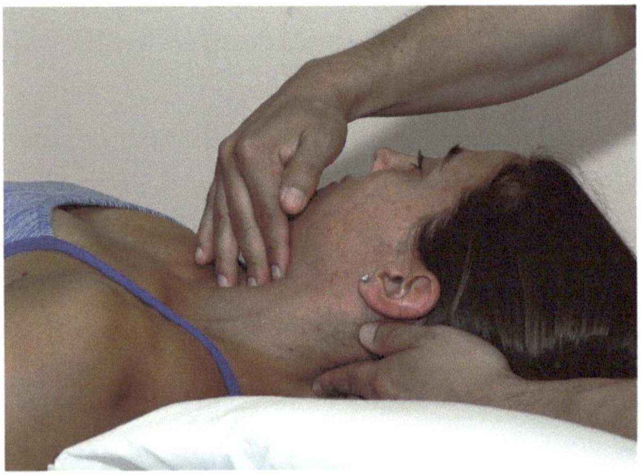

Typical fascial treatment to address cervical fascial structures.

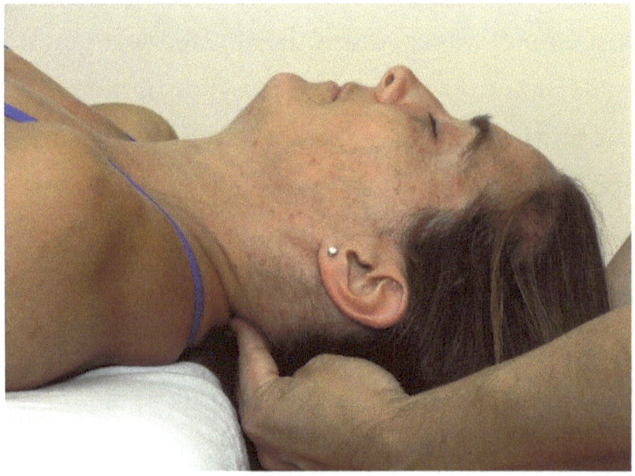

When caution is needed, the structures can also be targeted via the positional work of SCS.

Other conditions such as surgeries, surgical implants, or personal apprehensions make the use of SCS preferable. There's also one skill I have observed in therapists proficient in SCS, and that is having the ability to sense how far, and in what directions, the body wants to unwind to release the targeted dysfunction. The more accomplished therapists understand the enormous value of the SCS methodology and won't hesitate to use it as circumstances justify.

Although I will be emphasizing the fascial model since it's the one that I use almost exclusively in my practice, the soul of Counterstrain remains the same. It is my intent to focus on the power and efficiency of Fascial Counterstrain while remaining respectful of the original work. It is, after all, what helped me identify the vicious cycle in pain therapy.

THE VICIOUS CYCLE IN PAIN THERAPY

I have a mission in life: To help you live a joyous, energized, and pain-free life.

While the means of delivery have changed, the core mission has not. It is this yearning that drove me from the technology field to strength and wellness, and ultimately pain therapy.

My curiosity for the strength field was sparked by legendary strongmen. One of my most vivid childhood memories is that of Soviet weightlifter Vasily Alekseyev on TV as he shattered world records. The ease and elegance in which this mighty Olympian became the first human ever to put over 500 pounds overhead in competition left me astonished and made a lasting impression.

But the one who made me realize that strength was a lifestyle was my Dad. My typical childhood drawings of him depicted him performing his calisthenics and martial-arts drills. As an accomplished martial artist, marathon runner, and aspiring bodybuilder, he taught us by example of the freedom and joy that strength and fitness bring to life.

And it was this joy and freedom what led me out of the technology field. Seeing how I would escape the stress of the day on the exercise floor, I decided I'd use my savings, apply for scholarships, and get student loans to return to school and pursue my degree in Exercise Science.

The more I learned, the more I applied, and the more I discovered, the more my joy and spirits were elevated. The exercise floor never failed to bring me peace. And I wanted everyone to experience that elation—the clarity of mind that comes after completing a challenging workout, the sweetness of mastering a new skill, and the powerful energy that vibrates deep inside us and dons us confidence, gracefulness, and an assertive demeanor.

My drive for learning and improvement earned me a solid reputation, a full appointment book, and the privilege of being featured in popular media. I felt unstoppable.

target training

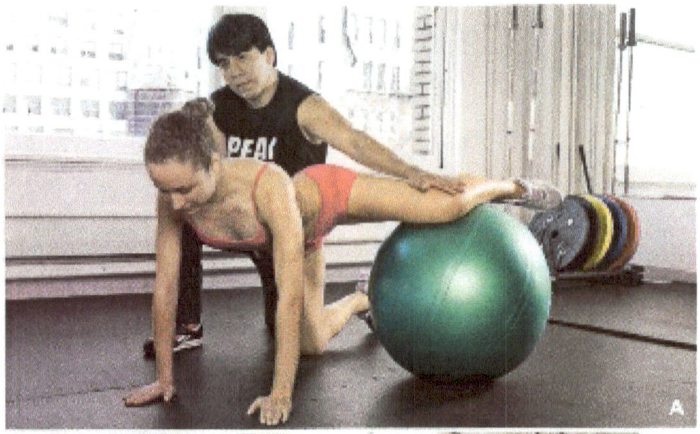

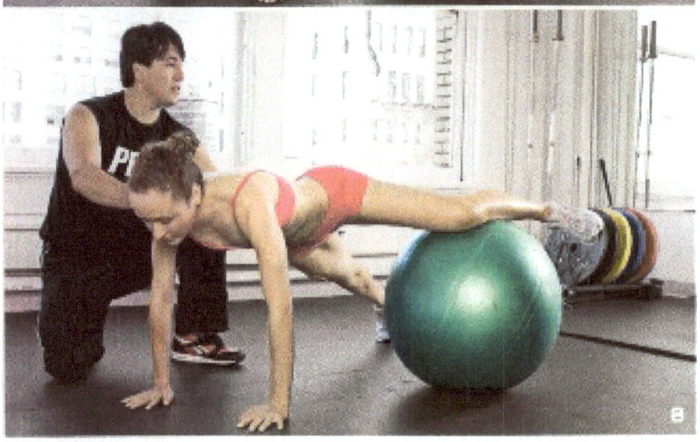

thigh circle

Works inner thighs and core

> Grab a stability ball and kneel on all fours, wrists aligned with shoulders and knees under hips. Raise left knee out to side to hip height and rest inside of knee on center of ball [A].

> Press knee onto ball and keep abs tight and head in line with spine as you straighten right leg [B]. Find your balance, then make small clockwise circles with the ball.

> Do 16 to 20 circles, then switch legs to complete set. Do 2 sets; make counterclockwise circles during the second set.

> Trainer's tip
A wider stance makes the move easier. Keep it narrow for the biggest challenge.

YOU CAN DO THESE AT HOME, TOO

You'll need a resistance band and a stability ball or ottoman (find exercise equipment at *shapeupshop.com*).

> Lateral resisted squat Do it with a resistance band looped around your waist and attached to a sturdy object.

> Step-up and knee raise Try this move with a resistance band looped around your thigh and attached to a sturdy object.

> Thigh circle If you don't have a stability ball, do the move with your knee on an ottoman (one with wheels is best).

take it up a notch

Advanced exercisers should add weight and/or follow these special instructions.

advanced program

what to do	lateral resisted squat	step-up and knee raise	thigh circle
sets	3 or 4	3 or 4	2
reps	8	8	16–20
weight range	up to 50 pounds	same	n/a
special instructions	Adding weight is enough of a challenge.	Let go of the Body Bar or hold the knee raise for 2 to 3 counts.	Raise your balancing leg off the floor.

From Shape Magazine, July 2007, Volume 26, No. 11, Pages 134-138.

How the Cycle Goes

Had you asked me then if I ever saw myself in the manual therapy medicine field, I would've snickered. What insanity would justify leaving the spotlight, the accolades, and the enormous satisfaction for something so irrelevant?

The answer would soon arrive in the form of the frustration I'd face as injuries trapped me in the vicious cycle of big efforts producing meager results and eventually a relapse. While at first I'd blame myself or thought of me as an anomaly, I'd eventually discover that more people shared my predicament.

Take for instance, a common scenario in which a healthy individual's minor back pain turned into an unbearable ordeal after something as mundane as bending over to tie their shoes.

"It's a herniated disc," the experts had said. "That's what happens when you bend at the waist." But the imaging studies did not support the diagnosis [6] [7] [8].

The confused patient then consulted a new expert who determined that the problem was a weak core. The solution? Strengthen it!

But core strengthening did little and even exacerbated the pain [9]. "You're doing the exercises wrong!" the core expert admonished, urging the patient to correct their faulty form.

When the corrections brought more frustration than relief, the patient switched to a new expert and learned that the problem was never the discs or the core, but an unstable sacroiliac (SI) joint, which the expert fixed to provide relief.

It all went smoothly for about a month when, out of nowhere, the back flared up again. So, the patient returned to the SI joint expert, but this time the relief only lasted a couple of weeks. Further treatments delivered even shorter-lasting results until treating the SI joint no longer provided relief.

The concerned patient then resumed searching, baffled by the conflicting opinions. One expert told them it was their posture but working at correcting posture did little to mitigate the pain [10]. That was because the movement expert, not the posture expert, had the answers. According to the movement expert, the pain was the result of the patient's faulty motor patterns, so the patient had to learn how to make sure their glutes fired, their quads and hamstring were in harmonious ratios [11], their multifidi stabilized, and their pelvic floor engaged.

But when results were, at best, marginal, the patient learned from the myofascia expert that the problem was a tight iliopsoas. And not only did the myofascia expert release the iliopsoas but also taught the patient how to release their quads, hamstrings, glutes, and piriformis via challenging self-applied techniques and stretches, all of which were touted as crucial to avoid relapsing.

Thus, the patient worked hard every day to make sure their glutes fired, their pelvic floor, multifidi, and scapulae engaged, and that they were walking with perfect mechanics, perfect posture, and engaging the transversus abdominis because... core! In addition, they had to be diligent about their supplements, daily stretching, and use of rollers, balls, and other devices designed to tame stubborn muscles.

Little by little the patient started feeling relief but deep inside, they also felt that something still lurked, something that could set them back should they neglect their complex routines. Yet the hesitation faded as they made more progress and thought that, perhaps, it was possible to regain a pain-free life after all.

That is, until they bent over to tie their shoes and threw their backs out again.

Breaking the Vicious Cycle

Was the previous scenario too outlandish? I wish I could say so but it is a compendium of multiple experiences, including my own. But occasionally, fortune smiles upon the right person and the circumstances work to break the vicious cycle and spare them further aggravation.

One of such circumstances took place in the spring of 2014, as one of the participants in my exercise class was slowed down by knee pain. He revealed that his knee had been bothering him for months after single-leg squats, and how frustrated he was with the lack of progress. I asked if he had a formal diagnosis and he mentioned that despite all the negative studies, he had been diagnosed with a torn meniscus.

But I had seen this gentleman move, and I had experience treating torn menisci. His patterns were not of a typical meniscus tear so I asked if he didn't mind that I took a look. He gave me the go-ahead and, with a skeptical smile, mentioned he was diagnosed by reputable orthopedists. My assessment revealed local vascular involvement, which I proceeded to clear.

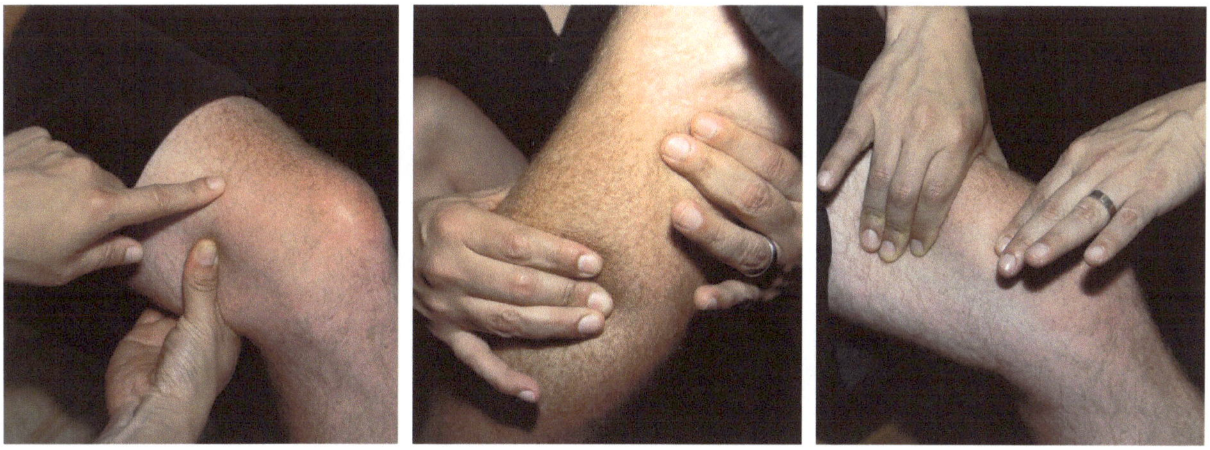

His full attention was on my work. He was curious at the gentleness of the maneuvers and even more curious that I had only mentioned vascular structures and not a single muscle or ligament. When he stood up, his dropping jaw and wandering eyes revealed what Counterstrain neophytes experience: *How's this even possible?*

He walked around and squatted with comfort, in awe of what a few minutes of work accomplished. As difficult as it was for him to accept the results, it was even more difficult to learn what had been driving his pain. *What do vascular structures have to do with pain? How do they move a joint anyway?*

And no, vascular structures are not the only ones that can affect the knee joint, but they're common. More often than not, due to the mechanics of the joint itself and the adjacent joints, there will be more than one structure or physiological system involved. Full function and health resume only when they're all identified and cleared.

Needless to say, he was both pleased and upset. He was enjoying the results from this fortuitous encounter, but not too thrilled that he had been stuck in the vicious cycle for so long. Having been there myself, I fully understand, but I also have deep sympathy for all therapists involved.

The most soul-crushing feeling for a therapist is the inability to help our clients despite our best efforts. It makes us doubt our skills, competence, and our calling. But this soul-crushing feeling can also be a driving force and guide us to new possibilities.

Not only was I the client who endured the frustrating vicious cycle, I was also the therapist who experienced heartbreaking frustration as his caseload grew more complex. But my mission was my fuel. The mission that made me embrace the strength and conditioning field was what made me transition from the training floor to the treatment table.

FROM THE TRAINING FLOOR TO THE TREATMENT TABLE

Prior to my involvement in manual therapy medicine, my devotion to the strength field knew no boundaries. I was convinced that as long as we cultivated our strength, our bodies would be injury-free. And, should the unpredictable temporarily put us out of commission, that we could easily reclaim it all through exercise.

This was the ideology that molded my views about manual therapy. Even though I knew that its roots were medicinal, I felt that it had deteriorated into an indulgence for the lazy and the feeble. My views of chiropractic manipulation were even less kind after a sour experience in college. To top it all, my own life experiences had reinforced my views as I got away with a lot. There was no such thing as a rest day for me. I passionately believed that if I cycled my loads and times properly, there was no need to take time off. The minor injuries I experienced were resolved after a few days of light activity, stretching, ice, and anti-inflammatories. I proudly reached my thirties without ever experiencing a disabling injury.

That all came to a screeching halt in October 2002, when life showed me how my zealotry had taken me away from the essence of my mission.

The Sigh at the Door

I felt nauseated and I broke into copious sweating.

I was barely able to rerack the heavy barbell I had been squatting as I prepared for a weight-lifting competition. A sudden pop in my back at the bottom of the exercise had stopped me with overwhelming pain. I rested my head on the barbell fighting dread and uncertainty, but I still managed to feign calmness. Deep inside, though, my entrails tightened and my heart raced as I tried to figure out what was going on.

After a few painful minutes of clearing the weights, I pretended to walk away casually but the noticeable limp betrayed me. I had never experienced pain that paralyzed my right hip and flank, sending fire and spasms down my leg.

For the first time in my life, the modalities I had used in the past proved useless and even produced more pain than relief.

Imaging studies revealed bulging discs at the lumbar spine. I was reassured that the protocol of epidural shots, physical therapy, and adequate rest would bring relief, but despite following all the therapeutic guidelines for six weeks, the relief never came. Other than some short-lived relief after ultrasound, the pain didn't budge.

When one of my friends who had recently been in agonizing back pain noticed me losing hope, he suggested what I had sworn off. "Go see this chiropractor," he said, handing me the card for Dr. Matt Cooper. "He's helped my back a lot," my friend said, making circles with his hips without pain. This proved a strong lure and in a matter of days, I found myself heading to Dr. Cooper's office. I sighed at his front door, recalling my previous chiropractic experience.

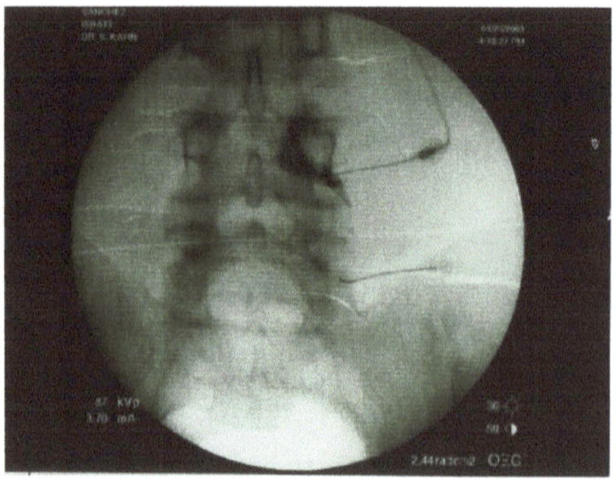

My first epidural shot. Circa February 2003

Hope in Manual Therapy Medicine

Dr. Cooper carefully studied the results from my medical images and procedures. Based on them, he designed a treatment plan that would help me heal without risking further injury.

Though his first treatment gave me a glimpse of hope, it wasn't enough to shake off my skepticism. Subsequent treatments helped a bit more, but not enough. It was then that my physiatrist started contemplating surgery and I felt tempted to comply.

Dr. Cooper advised me to think it carefully. At that point, I had gotten to know him better and realized that he understood his field well and was passionate about helping his patients. Unlike other healthcare professionals, Dr. Cooper believed that I would be able to return to all my activities—but I had to let my body heal first.

After a heart-to-heart conversation, Dr. Cooper suggested a discogram, as the unpleasant procedure was the most reliable method to determine whether the discs were driving the back pain. Much to my confusion, the painful test was negative, meaning my pain was not caused by the discs. But my physiatrist still wanted to go ahead with the surgery, and I was so fed up with the pain that I was ready to schedule it. But Dr. Cooper had another suggestion.

"Give me a shot," Dr. Cooper said. "Now that I know it's not the discs, I want to try something different. If you're still in pain after a few treatments, then you can get your surgery, but let me work on you first."

I agreed not because I had high hopes but because I wanted to prove that my only recourse was surgery. My mind clung to skepticism as Dr. Cooper placed me on his treatment table. This time, however, the treatment positions were different, and he was also treating different segments. The grand finale produced a loud pop … and my pain ceased immediately.

I didn't know what to say, or how to react.

For the first time in months my hips and legs felt strong and grounded, and I left his office without the limp that had accompanied me from the beginning of this incident. For the first time, I saw manual therapy in a different light and my skepticism for chiropractic medicine vanished. All the months of pain, invasive procedures, and expensive tests seemed like an unnecessary joke. Two more treatments was all I needed to regain my confidence and hope.

I contemplated manual therapy as the preferred pain solution not only for me but also for those who sought my expertise on the training floor. And no, I did not even remotely contemplate manual therapy medicine as a possible career path—I only wanted to return to the excitement of the training floor. Instead, I saw it as an invaluable ally in the path to wellness.

Catching my Attention

The lessons and wisdom from this incident were immensely helpful as I picked up a wave of clients who felt that, because of this injury, I could understand them better. That's when I started noticing parallels to my own experience. These folks would start their training with unmatched excitement, make rapid measurable progress, and then experience an unexplainable injury just as they were feeling their best.

There seemed to be no pattern. It didn't matter what preventive routines I'd develop. Even though the injuries happened to only a small group, I could not dismiss them as exceptions because there would be others just like them, and if I failed the initial group, I would also fail the newcomers.

My saving grace had been Dr. Cooper, but he had relocated. My only advice was to tell my clients to seek help from their own chiropractors to expedite their healing. That's when I started noticing another trend. Many of those who found relief would succumb to the same dysfunction in a few months. And there were those who experienced no relief at all.

Fortunately, my learning path was also steering my attention to the power of soft-tissue work. I had met a few accomplished bodyworkers specializing in ART, MAT, Rolfing, and other techniques. Having received excellent work from them in the absence of Dr. Cooper, I included them in my list of referrals.

In addition, many of my colleagues in the training field had started pursuing manual therapy education. The knowledge they were acquiring fascinated me and I wanted it, but I wanted it without getting involved. My time was just too precious.

Priceless Skills

My task was straightforward: create excellent training programs, ensure that my clients followed them properly, offset the possibility of injury with preventive measures, and have my colleagues studying manual therapy take care of their issues. My reputation grew and more people sought my services. I was happy!

Or was I?

I did enjoy the recognition, the referrals, and the friendships—yet I felt I was not serving to my full capacity. Something was missing, an unexplainable void that escaped all logic.

The answer soon materialized while observing one of my colleagues training one of his recreational athletes. In the middle of an agility-ladder drill, his client winced and verbalized his pain. He had not fallen or received impact, nor had his joints bent at an unnatural angle. Yet here he was, grimacing and noticeably limping. My colleague took him aside and applied the manual therapy techniques he had been learning. Much to my surprise, the athlete got up after a half-hour treatment and headed to the showers walking normally, all traces of pain and limping absent.

The ability to have those skills handy—ready to deliver prompt relief—was, indeed, powerful.

I was conflicted. Not having those skills in my arsenal felt irresponsible, but I tried to reason that my time was limited and I would be better off referring them to specialized therapists. Soon, the satisfaction I derived from the training floor started to dwindle.

This wasn't going to last long, though, for I was about to receive my next wake-up call.

The Cost of Stubbornness

One of my favorite summer events was the weightlifting camp organized by the East Coast Gold weightlifting team under the direction of USAW International Coach Leo Totten. What an amazing opportunity to get coaching from the top names in the sport, not to mention the camaraderie forged by improving our skills through grueling workouts.

Weightlifting camp in June 2007 found me preoccupied with my right knee. While I recognized that I had been lifting heavier weights, it wasn't by a margin large enough to justify the sporadic inflammation. Sometimes the knee would be fine with heavy lifting. Sometimes all it took to flare it up was a walk. I had debated whether to put the knee under such demands, but I was in the process of relocating to the Pacific Northwest and this would be my last weightlifting camp. I decided to go but I also decided that I'd be cautious and not get carried away.

The cautionary reluctance lasted but a day. I was feeling energized and though the knee would initially complain, its protest faded after the warmup. I even felt confident about setting new personal records. But on the third day the knee made its discontent more evident, and I finally decided to compromise. As I approached the barbell to execute a heavy clean, I decided I'd set a new personal record and then take it easy for the rest of camp.

The pain at the bottom of the receiving position made me drop the bar. The world slowed down as I watched the bar bounce and roll away.

"Are you okay?" my workout buddy asked.

His voice sounded muffled. I looked down at my knee, afraid of what I'd see but it looked normal. The sight brought me back.

"Dude, are you okay?" he asked again.

I was drenched in sweat and my heart raced. I straightened my knee and it complied, almost pain-free. I smiled.

"A tweak in my knee," I said, thinking I had been spared from a major injury.

Trying to get back on my feet made me realize that I hadn't. I was able to straighten my knee, but bending it proved painful, as did weight-bearing. While the knee didn't look deformed, that didn't mean it had not sustained a significant injury.

Ice and anti-inflammatories didn't do much to calm the pain. But, fortunately, my roommate and fellow weightlifter was pursuing manual therapy training. He applied deep-tissue techniques, and though I clenched my teeth during treatment, I could not deny that I experienced enough relief to sleep without disruption.

The morning after found me calmer and though the knee didn't look worse, it still couldn't bear weight. I went to see my physician in an emergency visit and though the X-Rays found no chips or fractures, he still wanted to be more thorough and gave me a prescription for an MRI and anti-inflammatories. The next steps would be determined by the MRI results.

Bitter Disappointments

"Four to five weeks," my doctor said, while going over the MRI images and report.

The partial tear in the patellar tendon reminded me of the folly of ignoring the warnings our bodies send us. But I was encouraged. That meant that by late July, at the latest, I'd be able to return to my activities. A physical therapist friend set me up with a rehab program, which I followed diligently, exercising, stretching, and icing as recommended—and sometimes more. Yet the pain didn't budge.

Five weeks passed and I was in as much discomfort as the when the injury happened. My concerned physician gave me a prescription for stronger anti-inflammatories and a referral to see one of the most touted orthopedists in the region, one who was supposedly so good that he frequently worked with professional sports teams.

I was excited and hopeful. I would finally find my answers.

Nah!

The orthopedist kept me waiting for over two hours, barely glanced at my knee, and dismissed all my questions. After ten minutes of poking and taking notes, he wrote me a prescription for physical therapy, more anti-inflammatories, and walked away.

My mood blinded me to the brightness of the late summer day. There was no way I'd be taking more anti-inflammatories. The stronger prescription my doctor had given me felt like two cats fighting in my entrails. This new prescription looked even more terrifying. And there was no way that a new physical therapy program would be different than what I had already.

My disappointment turned into anger as I swore off mainstream medicine, but then I also remembered what my roommate at weightlifting camp did. I had the fortune of having colleagues studying different manual therapy modalities, so I'd start there.

Manual Therapy to the Rescue

For the next month and half, manual therapy became an essential component of my healing, even when I occasionally doubted its effectiveness. Yet it was undeniable that—despite how the experts argued about their rationales and rarely came to a consensus—many people were healing through manual therapy.

I realized then how much I had closed myself to a unique educational opportunity. The least I could do was try the intro courses. If they were congruent with my mission, great! I'd have more invaluable assets. If they weren't, I'd no longer be tormented by the doubt.

Thus, October 2007 saw me at my first-ever manual therapy class, and my perspective of its role in my career completely changed. Was it the information? Partially. Rather, it was the application what made me see its potential.

I had arrived with my knee still in pain. Upon learning my story, one of the attendees worked on my injured leg at the end of the first day of class, and I experienced a relief I hadn't experienced in a while. I thought the relief would last only a day but the third and last day of class still found me without pain. Even after returning home, the knee still felt fine. I attempted exercises I had not attempted since my injury, and while I found stiffness, there was no pain.

Manual therapy had come to the rescue again, and this time, I could not ignore it.

The thought of incorporating manual therapy as an essential component of my strength training practice drew a smile and brought back the bliss that had long been missing. This was the right step in my path.

The Powerful Combination

The fulfillment and joy I was experiencing were at a much higher level. Having the ability to take care of my clients' injuries immediately cemented my mission and was a winning addition to my practice. My only regret was not having started sooner.

This was not an easy task. The year I chose to immerse in the manual therapy field was also the year I relocated to the Pacific Northwest and started new ventures. But my efforts paid off and soon, I earned an excellent reputation. Not only could I help you be in top shape, I could also dig in deep and reach those hard-to-get spots to treat your injuries—and while the treatment frequently proved uncomfortable, it also proved effective.

Soon, my appointment book was filling up with people who were more interested in pain therapy than in strength training. This was uncharted territory but all doubts vanished when I received a referral from a physician for a case of stubborn neck pain. To the surprise of the client and her physician, it took me only three sessions to eliminate it. This earned me more referrals and increased my desire to further my training. When I was able to resolve a thirty-five-year case of back pain in three weeks, I became the go-to guy.

One would think this would be the beginning of a streak of success stories, but life would soon bring its unpredictability when other physicians started sending me their pain cases.

This new batch was of different demographics. They didn't care about a healthy lifestyle or strength training, nor did they care about implementing them. They only wanted to deal with the pain interfering with their lives. These were the most challenging cases I had yet seen, and for the first time in my career as a pain therapist, I started meeting failure. It didn't matter what I did. The techniques that had brought relief to painful hips, backs, necks, knees, and shoulders were ineffective in this group.

How could this be when my skills were on the rise? The baffling cases kept arriving and I felt lost. How many times and in how many ways can one treat the same quadratus lumborum, latissimus dorsi, or splenius group, and expect a different result?

At that point I already knew of a therapist named Timothy Hodges whose practice was also in my then-hometown of Bainbridge Island, Washington, and who used a set of techniques tongue-twistingly called **Strain-Counterstrain**. Apparently, he was having success where even reputable therapists had failed.

The cases coming to my practice kept getting more complex, smacking my confidence and making me question my competence. One of them was a female in her mid-forties with a severe case of back pain. After six sessions of applying all I knew, I suggested she see Tim and to keep me posted.

A week later, her call baffled me. Tim had resolved her pain in only one session. What was it that Tim saw that I didn't? What did he do to resolve in one session what I couldn't even improve in six?

I've got to meet this guy, I thought as I browsed for his number.

THAT WAS NOT A MUSCLE

Tim Hodges graciously made time for me despite his busy schedule. I couldn't wait to meet him and settle the confusion that dazed me since my client called me.

In the meantime, I started to learn more about him. The degrees of separation in our small community meant that many of his clients were friends of my friends. The more I learned, the more perplexed I was. From individuals finding relief from Lyme disease symptoms, children returning to their energetic selves after experiencing what was considered severe trauma, or frozen shoulders impervious to other therapies—some of which I had overseen—these were the type of cases that would frustrate the medical community as well as manual therapists.

What can he see that the rest of us miss? All I could do was speculate.

Blasphemy!

I met with Tim at one of the local watering holes at the end of his day. I had planned to open with a friendly chat but my curiosity overwhelmed me and I started by inquiring about my client.

"So, what was her issue?" I asked.

"It was pretty straightforward, only one system," Tim said. "That's why her pain resolved quickly."

System? I thought. *As in…?* I had no idea what Tim had meant by *system*, nor did I have a frame of reference, so I steered the conversation back to my dimension. "So, which muscle was it, then?"

"That was not a muscle, it was a vein," Tim said, with the casualness of everyday news, looking at his drink menu, oblivious to my reaction.

My mind drew a blank, rendering me unable to produce words. What Tim had just said was blasphemy in the world of manual therapy medicine. Throughout all my training, it had been made clear that veins, arteries, nerves, and fossae were off-limits, and that there was no reason to go there. The consensus was that the aforementioned had no active role in musculoskeletal pain or dysfunction, thus the thought of manipulating them was fruitless and reckless. I couldn't even form a mental picture.

"A vein? How's that possible? How do you treat it?" I finally asked.

"Indirectly," Tim said.

My mind drew an even larger blank. It was the first time I heard the word *indirectly* applied to bodywork in a physical context.

"Indirectly?" I asked. "Is it like energy work or something similar?"

"Nothing like that." Tim chuckled.

He then proceeded to explain the relationship of veins, arteries, nerves, and organs in the deep fascial realm, their interactions, and how through gentle skilled manipulation the therapist could use one structure as a conduit to treat another. He told me of his success with Jones SCS, and also of his struggles as the cases got more complex, and how the advent of the fascial model was helping him in cases he'd normally get stuck. Over and over, he mentioned a name that would soon become an important one in my career: Brian Tuckey.

At that point, I didn't know who Brian was, nor had I heard of him, and I didn't feel like finding out more. I was only interested in physiological interactions and proof, and Tim Hodges was about to make me realize how little I actually knew.

When Anecdote Encounters Proof

I listened to Tim's every word. The information he was delivering was new to me—and challenging. Though my therapeutic repertoire included organ work, my attention was directed to the musculoskeletal system. Up to that very moment, I thought it was all we needed to treat pain and dysfunction. Yet Tim was sharing knowledge that shattered these concepts.

I thought I'd save face by mentioning my success cases via organ treatment. I thought I had finally gotten Tim's attention after I mentioned how I was able to unlock a frozen shoulder by treating the liver. But Tim was only curious and asked me what part of the liver I had treated.

"The whole liver," I said, not knowing what he meant. "Does it matter what part?"

"It does," Tim said. "Where did you do most of the work?"

I drew a blank again. "I'm not quite sure what you mean."

Tim smiled. "Was it the triangular ligament or the falciform ligament? Or did your work affect the common bile duct? Maybe you had an effect on the hepatic or portal veins?"

I felt the heat and flushness on my face. I hadn't even heard about half of the structures. All I could do was shrug.

"I didn't even know you could work those parts," I admitted.

"It's different with Counterstrain," Tim said.

We continued our conversation on the evolution of his practice, the modalities he had studied, and we started talking about remarkable cases. It was then that I recalled a case I had seen in his blog. This case was so extraordinary that it had been shared countless times on social media [12]. When I asked, Tim browsed his cell phone for the pictures.

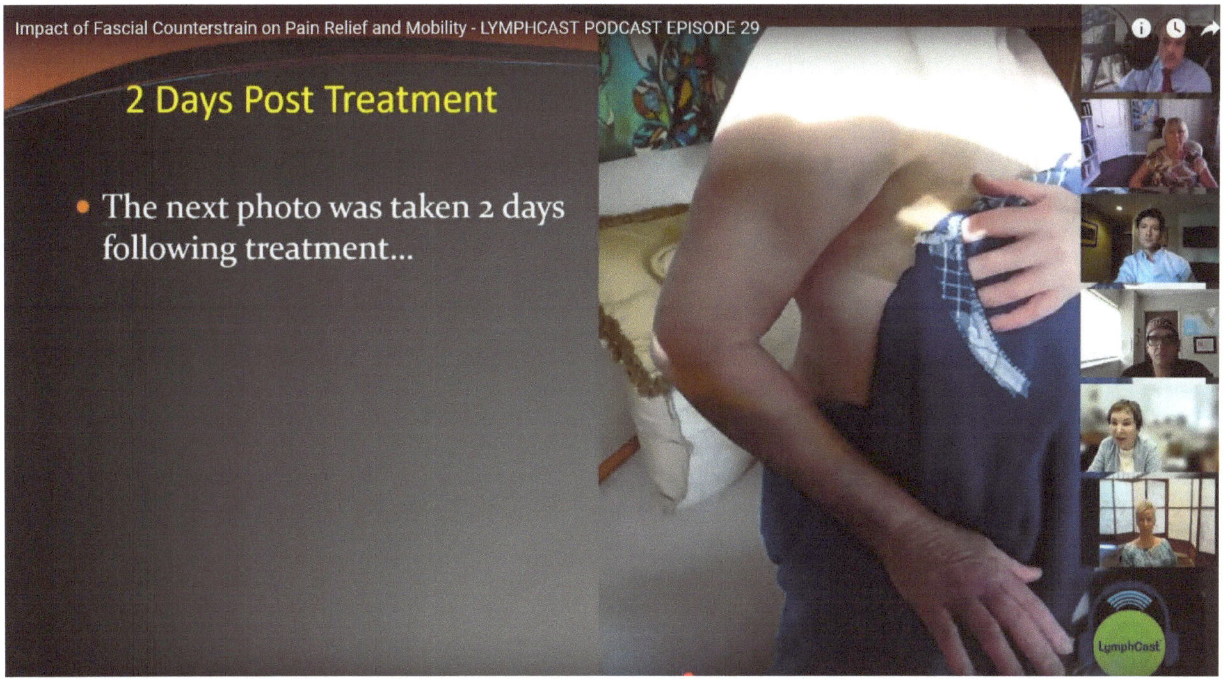

Brian Tuckey shares the details of Tim's case in episode 29 of the LymphCast Podcast. What I love most about the video is the genuine reaction from attendees as Brian reveals the aftermath of FCS therapy.

It was one thing seeing the pictures and reading the article in his blog, and a whole different game seeing the pictures in their full resolution and hearing Tim himself go over the case and his approach.

The client in question had sustained a hard fall that resulted in a mild fracture to the head of her humerus and was in so much pain that she couldn't move the entire right upper extremity. The client had been given prescriptions and a sling but they provided little relief.

At the insistence of her acquaintances, she went to see Tim but her pain, sling, and apprehension made it difficult for him to perform a complete evaluation. Tim could only guess the severeness of the damage s by the black, green, and yellowish discoloration in her hand—the only visible part of her affected limb.

Tim then showed me the *Before* picture in its full brutality and explained that it wasn't the damaged tissue that caused the uncontrolled swelling and the pain, but rather, the spasms—or aberrant reflex arcs—that blocked the retuning pathways of the lymphatic/venous systems and prevented the area from draining. That's what directed him to apply FCS techniques for vascular structures of the upper thorax—which I never thought were relevant in manual therapy.

Tim then showed me the *After* picture, taken a few days post-treatment by the client's spouse. Even though I had seen the pictorial comparison in Tim's blog, there was something about being in front of the therapist responsible for such a miracle. Perhaps it was the fact that this was now tangible and no longer anecdotal, an event in which those involved could be easily reached. Tim noticed my stupefaction and confided that the results also took him by surprise since he hadn't seen the true extent of the damage until then.

I needed no more convincing. My heart longed for such incredible skills and knowledge.

"This is stuff blows my mind," I said. "I really want to learn it—how do I go about it?"

Tim fixed his eyes on me and, without blinking, he asked: "Are you willing to unlearn what you've been taught?"

It was an honest and intense question. This meeting had already created doubts about what I thought were infallible facts but had also given me a clarity I had not experienced in a while. Tim guided me as to what courses to take and in what order, and if I so desired, to contact him for his Counterstrain mastery program after completing any of the modules.

The next introductory course would not be offered in my area until April 2012. I would use the time to review anatomy and fine-tune my manual therapy skills.

April 2012 could not arrive fast enough.

That Day in April 2012

The sun teased with its presence the Friday of the last weekend of April 2012, with a feeling akin to the restlessness of Christmas Eve as it transitions into Christmas day. I was part of a group of therapists taking their first steps into the fascinating world of Strain-Counterstrain (SCS) under the guidance of Larry Ham and Tim Hodges.

It wasn't like anything I had learned or been exposed to before. From joint motion-testing to the localization of tender points, and the application of the appropriate technique—it was all a game of precision and finesse. A couple of millimeters off in positioning and the release of the affected structure would cease. A couple of millimeters off in palpation and we'd be monitoring a completely different tender point, which in turn would not respond to the intended treatment.

What was even more astounding was feeling problem areas and hypertonic tissues virtually disappear at my fingertips. No need for heavy kneading. I thought of those clients I had to turn away because my direct deep tissue work would be too much for them—and how Strain-Counterstrain could help them.

Onward with the Journey

I took the second SCS module only two weeks after the first one. I had been practicing and studying but I was still having a hard time making sense of it. But I had no choice. I had already committed my time and resources, and all I could do was press on.

Thankfully, I had a three-month respite until the third SCS module so I had plenty of time to practice before adding new material. And practice I did, not only to master the method, but also because I was conflicted. I had been mixing postural assessments with SCS tender point identification to narrow down my findings but, time and time again, the findings from the methodologies rarely matched.

A shoulder rotated anteriorly used to mean that I should give attention to the pectoralis group and the latissimus, and if that failed, I should work on the lungs. But quite often, SCS testing would indicate that while the shoulder was rotated anteriorly, it wasn't restricted, and that the structures that were jammed were the adjacent ribs. Applying SCS techniques for the lateral aspect of the ribs would resolve the dysfunction in two minutes and change the postural measurements not only on the shoulder, but also on the neck and pelvis.

As if that were not enough, there were times in which the affected structures and the postural conclusions matched. Whenever this happened, the structures would respond more to my direct deep tissue techniques rather than SCS. From time to time, the dysfunction would respond to neither.

I attributed this inconsistency to my newness compounded with missing a set of techniques. Knowing that I would soon take the third module gave me hope. In addition, I had already enrolled in Tim's Counterstrain Mastery program and we'd be going over the first module in extensive detail and lots of supervised practice under his experienced eyes.

I thought I'd have plenty to work on in 2012 but soon I'd be reconsidering that thought.

The Peak of Frustration

That suffocating feeling we experience when our best efforts are not enough? That feeling that disrupts our sleep and immerses our minds in myriad thoughts as we search for answers?

That feeling is frustration.

But frustration is not necessarily bad. Frustration is what makes us realize that the answers we seek are not where we are seeking, and that we must reach for new dimensions if we want to find them. It was frustration that first led me to the manual therapy medicine field, it was frustration what led me to Strain-Counterstrain (SCS), and it was frustration what drove me to add to my already packed education calendar.

Mid-July of 2012 saw my wife experience a back injury that resulted in pain she had never endured before. I didn't think much of it at first. I had helped countless cases of back pain, and she, being fit and in good health, looked to be routine treatment. But I was wrong—very wrong.

I applied all I knew and did all I could. All my direct deep tissue techniques, all the relevant SCS techniques—none made a difference. I had worked on my wife for seven sessions and while she occasionally reported a slight improvement, she'd relapse quickly and I'd not be able to reproduce the fleeting relief, even if I applied the same techniques. To make matters worse, I was heading out of town for five days on a trip I could not postpone. I decided, then, that this case was beyond my skills, and I contacted my friend Dhyana Moyer, an experienced Counterstrain Therapist, for help.

When I called my wife later on, she reported tremendous relief from her session with Dhyana. That night, my wife was able to finally sleep without being disrupted by pain and kept improving as the days went by. She was pretty much back to her energetic self when she picked me up upon my return.

I then contacted Dhyana to thank her for the miracle, for her skill and kindness, and to find out what SCS techniques she had applied. Dhyana reported that her work had been mostly Fascial Counterstrain (FCS) for the viscera and a tiny bit of work for the lymphatic/venous system.

I was in awe of the results from the visceral work, and as much as I wanted to rush and register for the next visceral course, I remembered that my plate was already full. Would it be prudent to add another course on top? In addition, my educational budget had already been taxed. It wouldn't be wise to start building debt at that point.

I decided that I would put all my efforts and focus on the third module and the mastery program. I would build a level of proficiency that would serve me well in my practice and in all upcoming courses.

Immersing in Counterstrain

August rolled in and so did the third module of SCS. Though I was still mixing tender point identification with postural measurements, I was treating all my cases mostly via SCS. I could not wait for the gems I'd add from this class.

The third module was taught by the then-director of the Jones Institute, Randy Kusunose. The emphasis was on SCS treatment for the cranium and, and of all the modules, this one carried the most mystery. It was astonishing to watch Randy release dysfunctions in the thorax and extremities by treating tender points in the head.

This was the class I enjoyed the most, maybe because the now-familiar company of other therapists enhanced the learning experience. In addition, many of the attendees were seasoned practitioners retaking the course to sharpen their skills. From them I heard again about Fascial Counterstrain and Brian Tuckey, of the fascial courses they had taken, and how life-changing they had been in their practices.

Only a few weeks after the third module, I—and a few other eager practitioners—started the mastery program under the guidance of Tim Hodges. Week after week he'd fine-tune our assessment skills, palpatory skills, and technique. A bonus for training with Tim was that he was exposed to the latest Counterstrain developments, and while he could not teach them to us, he could give us a demonstration. It was through the mastery program that I briefly witnessed the application of the cranial scan, and the precision and speed of Fascial Counterstrain (FCS).

I was curious and conflicted. FCS made sense and the ability to release a dysfunction via a gentle glide in less than a minute was a welcome and logical change. *But the cranial scan?* How did this witchy-sounding element even make it into the modality? Yet part of me recalled my conversations with practitioners who had already received fascial training and I realized that I was again rejecting an invaluable asset just because I thought it eccentric. I also recalled how Dhyana had helped my wife after my streak of treatment failures that included what I then knew of SCS.

I checked the Jones Institute website and found out that there were a couple of spots left for the FCS visceral class in Portland, Oregon, in a few weeks. I was flooded by a mix of urgency and confusion. This would be a significant investment of funds, time, and energy. I had already exceeded my educational budget for the year. I was already busy practicing what I had learned, attending the mastery program, and building a business. Was I spreading myself too thin?

I met with Tim Hodges to go over my conundrum. After a few pensive minutes, he nodded.

"I think you can handle it," he said. "It'll be a great addition, and we'll review it in the next mastery module."

That was all the encouragement I needed. I didn't quite know how I'd afford the expenses but in my heart I knew that waiting longer to discover fascial treatment was no longer an option.

Mind ... Blown!

I'll never forget the weekend of November 2–4, 2012 in Portland. I would finally get to meet Brian Tuckey, the creator of the fascial system, and learn from him about the application of Counterstrain principles on visceral structures.

My attention was fully engaged from the very first minute of the opening lecture. So many breakthroughs, so many *a-ha!* moments, but even greater revelations were about to materialize when Brian asked for a volunteer to start the practical segment. About a half dozen therapists, including yours truly, raised our hands.

Brian proceeded to place his hands on the first candidate's head, touching different cranial regions with certain but fast palpation. "Nope, you're arterial," Brian said, immediately moving on to the second candidate. He repeated the maneuver. "Nope, you're neural."

I watched him, fascinated by his ability to determine the involved system in a matter of seconds. When he arrived at me, he placed his fingers on the superior aspects of my mastoid processes—the pointy bones just behind and underneath the ear canals. The unexpected pain made me wince.

"Ooh, these are nasty!" Brian said, attempting to wiggle the rigid structures. "You're perfect."

Brian proceeded with the treatment for the tender points that represented different anchors of the pleura (the inner lining of the rib cage), the pericardium (the sac of connective tissue that envelops the heart) and other fascial structures of the cardio-respiratory system.

This was radically different from what I had given, received, and been exposed to. For the initial treatment which targeted the upper portion of the pleura, Brian simply applied a mild compression on the upper part of my chest and moved the segment upward. After thirty seconds, the tender point was no more, and I could feel the difference, all without any positional adjustments.

Brian continued by treating other areas in the rib cage, clearing the dysfunctions that affected their pertinent fascia. After completing the series, he returned to the mastoid processes. It was softer and painless to the touch, and as a bonus, I could also breathe better.

"Your lab partner will clear the rest," Brian said, patting my shoulder as he turned around to supervise the rest of the class. He never noticed my stupefaction as I tried to process what I had just been through. Further, the cranial scan proved its accuracy as a method of assessment. This was a completely different world of Counterstrain.

For the next three days, I practiced palpating the different areas of the cranial scan for dysfunctions in the visceral system, clearing them via gentle techniques, and confirming the effectiveness of the treatment in the corresponding cranial scan segment. The results were almost immediate and satisfying. I drew immense inspiration from watching Brian perform complete scans in a matter of seconds. I vowed then to take every available FCS module and to practice the cranial scan relentlessly.

Its Evolution is my Evolution

The FCS visceral module of the Counterstrain Mastery program launched with great energy in January 2013. Tim challenged us as he demanded palpatory precision and a high level of anatomical knowledge. Under his guidance and patience, our skills grew exponentially with each practice session.

There was also a new element in this mastery module: Clinical days.

Tim had made it clear that the only way to truly master Counterstrain was to apply it in the real world. The second half of the module included a clinical hour, where we treated real cases, folks who had volunteered for this work. We were allowed to use all the techniques we knew, and we could even use our manuals. But we wouldn't be all by ourselves. Tim would be close by, supervising and guiding.

It was sobering to see how much I had learned, equally sobering to see how much more I had to learn, and far more sobering to see how much I had to let go of. It became evident during the first clinical. I had reviewed my client's history and chief complaint. I was ready! Or was I?

The clients walked in directly to their assigned therapists. All my colleagues had them get comfortable on the treatment tables as they asked additional questions.

Not me.

I had mine stand against the wall as I asked questions and took measurements of neck, shoulder, and hip alignments. I also checked for asymmetry in rotations, for deviations in the cranial bones, and possible leg-length inequality. I was focused on my task until Tim tapped my shoulder and took me aside.

"I understand that this is how you normally assess," Tim said. "But we only have one hour and you've already spent ten minutes with your client against the wall."

I paid attention to my surroundings. Everyone was deeply involved in treatment. Many of the clients on the other treatment tables were already dozing off. I realized, then, that something had to change.

"You know enough to help your client," Tim said. "Trust the process. The rest will fall in place if you do your job correctly."

My heart pounded. I had never completed a treatment session relying exclusively on Counterstrain methods and the cranial scan. I had no choice but to press on but to my relief, my client's cranial scan revealed several visceral fascia dysfunctions.

All my practicing paid off as I was able to quickly identify and release structures without consulting the manual. Soon, I was all caught up and the visceral scan was changing remarkably.

Tim had also been right. The asymmetries and structural distortions I had initially observed were disappearing without my direct intervention. Treatment of the visceral ligamentous structures of the lower abdomen corrected pelvic rotation, inflare, and even the leg-length difference. The scan then shifted to the upper body and visceral treatment for the thorax released her shoulders, tight neck, and pain in the upper back—dysfunctions she had not reported because her lower back had consumed her full attention.

That was a pivotal point. I had been contemplating transitioning exclusively to the Counterstrain methodology but every time I wanted to do so, I hesitated. All this changed after that clinical day.

I continued taking classes and the Counterstrain Mastery modules offered by Tim. Reviewing the extensive material under his guidance proved to be one of the best investments I made in my education. Thanks to Tim, my palpatory skills and understanding of the method reached a level that allowed me to ace the Counterstrain Proficiency Test in October 2013. I didn't know I've had the highest score until Brian Tuckey announced it at the first-ever FCS Neural module in February of 2014 in San Diego.

Fast-forward to the present. I've taken virtually every module available and keep retaking them since the material keeps getting updated. All my work keeps paying off and now I find myself as part of a small group who has successfully passed the rigorous certification process and are officially certified as Fascial Counterstrain therapists (CSC I). In addition, I am also guiding other aspiring FCS therapists as a Teaching Assistant (TA) during the regular Jones Institute courses, which allows me to master the material at a deeper level.

FCS keeps evolving and I keep evolving along—its evolution is my evolution. I get an immense sense of purpose, hope, and enjoyment when I contemplate what's coming, what's getting discovered, and what's getting refined. I'm truly living my mission.

I invite you now to continue exploring our field and experience how, even though it feels like magic, the magic can be explained by solid scientific principles.

Let us now explore the nuts and bolts of Fascial Counterstrain.

It is impossible for a man to learn what he thinks he already knows.

EPICTETUS

THE NUTS AND BOLTS OF FASCIAL COUNTERSTRAIN

For all the mind-blowing and speedy results that this *indirect* method delivers with such finesse and gentleness to even the most complex conditions, one would think that FCS addresses phantasmal aspects of our physiology. One would even conjure images of obscure knowledge available only to a chosen cadre already beset with extraordinary powers.

While that idea is miles off target, I'll admit that FCS appears unconventional because rather than focusing on any particular anatomical structure as the sole driver of pain and dysfunction, FCS operates from where the responses governing pain and dysfunction converge and interact. This approach is the product of extensive research in the multiple branches of science investigating complex pain and dysfunction. While all these branches produce excellent works and breakthroughs, rarely do they venture outside their professional confines.

Ultimately, it was Brian Tuckey who dedicated thousands of hours to go over all the valuable research and put the pieces of the puzzle together. The end result is a trainable manual therapy system based on the one universal principle established by the late Dr. Jones:

Follow the direction of ease.

Since this direction of ease is actually a direction of decompression dictated by autonomic mechanisms, its path is not capricious or random. As long as we, as therapists, honor its governing physiological principles, our treatment will be painless and fruitful. Finding resistance means we're being forceful, or that our assessment and/or location are incorrect.

Prior to the summer of 2021, had you asked me what those governing physiological principles were, I would've told you that they were aberrant protective reflex arcs [3] affecting the fascial networks and that following the direction of ease was how we shut them off. That's no longer the case. While the answer was correct, it was not complete.

What is Fascial Counterstrain?

Defining the essence of FCS was not easy. We knew we were shutting off aberrant reflexes but it was difficult to explain how without resorting to heavy scientific language. Trying to explain what perpetuated their intrusive presence was even more complicated.

That all changed on August 22, 2021, when Brian's years of research were summarized in the paper "*Impaired Lymphatic Drainage and Interstitial Inflammatory Stasis in Chronic Musculoskeletal and Idiopathic Pain Syndromes*," which was officially published in *Frontiers in Pain Research*. In this paper, Brian presents a novel hypothesis that identifies a potential driving factor in the creation and perpetuation of chronic pain and dysfunction.

This in turn, allowed a theoretical rationale to emerge which made a plain-language definition possible. So, when we are asked, *What is Fascial Counterstrain?* we can say:

> *"Fascial Counterstrain is a complex process that identifies and removes trapped inflammation from all tissues in the body. The technique uses specific tender points to identify the location of inflammation which may impact any tissue in the body including muscles, ligaments, nerves, organs, or blood vessels."*

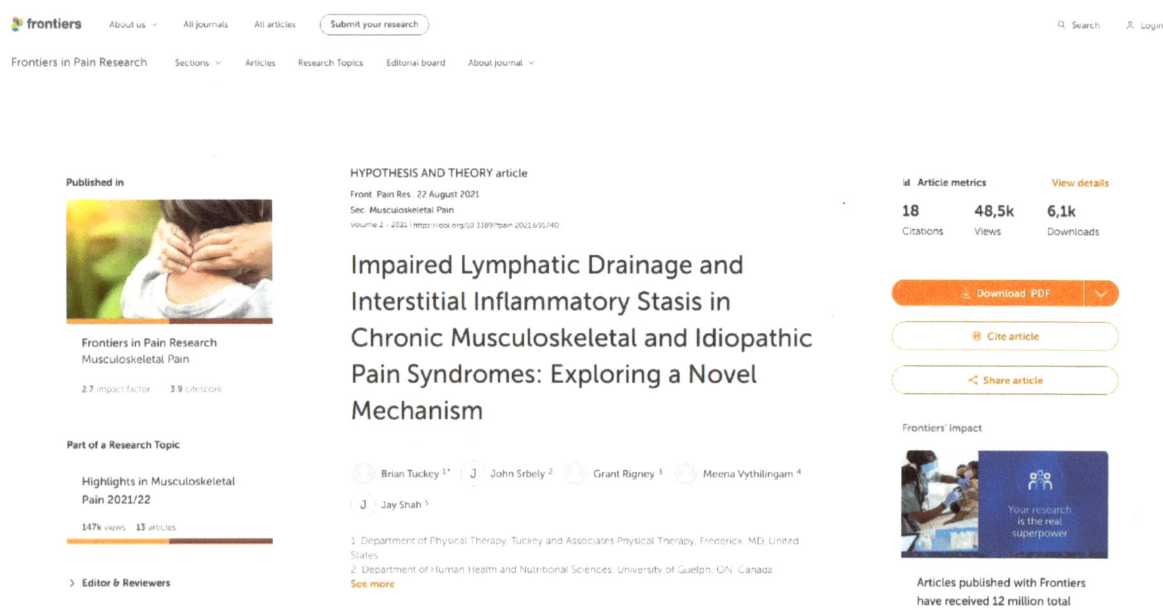

The aforementioned did not change the fact that we are still shutting off aberrant reflexes, but we no longer have to go on lengthy, multidimensional, anatomical explanations. Instead, we can now direct our attention to a more relatable outcome: *draining the trapped inflammation perpetuating the condition* [13].

You can access the article via the QR code, or the link below.

frontiers

HYPOTHESIS AND THEORY article

Front. Pain Res., 22 August 2021

Sec. Musculoskeletal Pain

Volume 2 - 2021 | https://doi.org/10.3389/fpain.2021.691740

Impaired Lymphatic Drainage and Interstitial Inflammatory Stasis in Chronic Musculoskeletal and Idiopathic Pain Syndromes: Exploring a Novel Mechanism

frontiersin.org/journals/pain-research/articles/10.3389/fpain.2021.691740/full

The direction of ease, or decompression, in our techniques is what creates the pressure gradient that allows the body to drain the trapped inflammation [14], which in turn is at the genesis of the many complex issues we see in our practices. Understanding that the myriad symptoms typical in pain and dysfunctions are potential expressions of autonomic defensive mechanisms, a.k.a. reflexes, resulting from trapped inflammation is what makes FCS so powerful.

Before exploring the mechanisms, I need to remind you that I'm condensing them to their more relevant aspects to convey the core concepts, but you may still need to go over the material a few times to connect all the components. I've also created blog posts that incorporate video to explain the mechanisms in more detail. You can access them at:

healing-and-strength.com/blog

And search for the *That was not a Muscle* tags for the relevant posts.

However, if you feel the details presented here are overly simplified and you desire a more in-depth explanation, then I invite you to explore the citations I've included.

What We All Know Happens

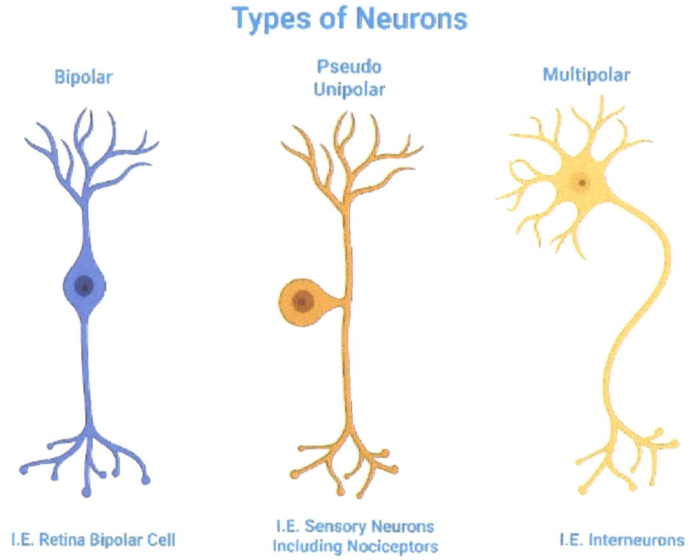

Every single structure in our bodies is loaded with sensory **nerve cells** or **neurons**. There are also motor neurons but we'll start by focusing on the **sensory neurons** since they monitor mechanical tension, temperature, biochemistry, and the subsequent disruptions to any of those factors [15]. Their signals go towards the spine or Central Nervous System (CNS), which makes them *afferent* units.

The sensory neurons that perceive pain are known as **nociceptors** as they detect painful and injurious stimuli [16].

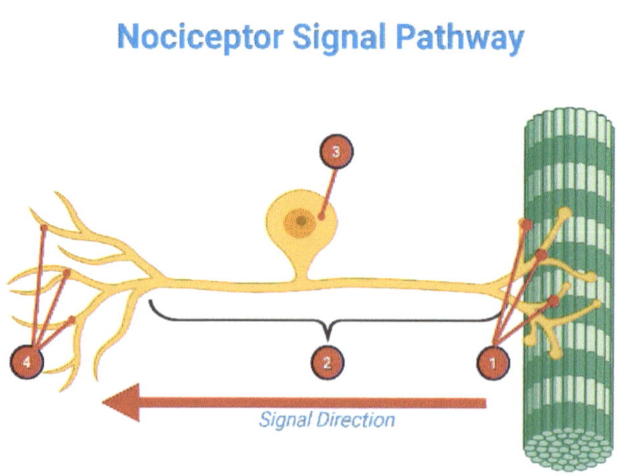

1) Nociceptor nerve endings connected to muscles, bones, arteries, veins, nerves, and all of our anatomical structures detect an injurious stimulus and turn it into a pain signal.

2) The pain signal travels through axon, the elongated part of the neuron toward the spine.

3) Signal gets processed at the nociceptor cell body/nucleus.

4) Signal continues to the nociceptor dendrites connecting to the deeper spinal structures.

Though we will be referring to the *primary—or peripheral—afferent nociceptors* for our purposes, there's a slight technical distinction between *primary afferent nociceptors* and just *nociceptors*. For simplicity, we'll be referring to all of them as *nociceptors*. Also, since these neurons are the first in the sensory upstream sequence, they're categorized as **first order neurons**.

There are four types of nociceptors classified by their velocity of conduction, but it's the **type III** and **IV** that are the most abundant in all fascial expressions. [17] You may have noticed that I use the term *fascial expression*, and that is because the whole of fascia is far more than myofascia.

In fact, the Foundation of Osteopathic Research and Clinical Endorsement (FORCE) has given us a more encompassing view, which is presented in Brian's paper. Fascia is, then,

> *"... Any tissue that contains features capable of responding to mechanical stimuli. The fascial continuum is the result of the evolution of the perfect synergy among different tissues, liquids, and solids, capable of supporting, dividing, penetrating, feeding, and connecting all the districts of the body: epidermis, dermis, fat, blood, lymph, and lymphatic vessels, the tissue covering the nervous filaments (endoneurium, perineurium, epineurium), voluntary striated muscle fibers and the tissue covering and permeating it (epimysium, perimysium, endomysium), ligaments, tendons, aponeurosis, cartilage, bones, meninges, involuntary striated musculature and involuntary smooth muscle (all viscera derived from the mesoderm)" [13] [17]*

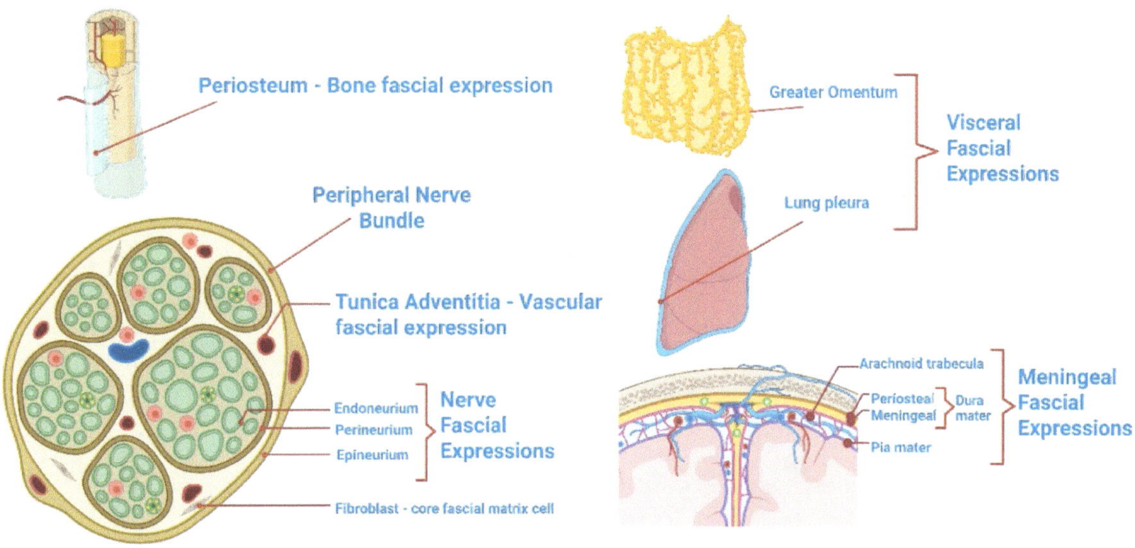

All of the aforementioned structures are fascia and as such, rich in type III and IV nociceptors, which makes them equally susceptible and reactive to disruptive environments and mechanisms, including all stages of injuries and injury healing. We can start by illustrating a typical **protective reflex arc**—the most immediate and automatic injury response—with an incident most of us have experienced: spraining our ankle.

Signal to Spine and Protection

The moment that sensory neurons in the ankle joint detect the abrupt disruption of tissue mechanics and tissue damage, they send signals that travel through their **axons** (the elongated portion of the neurons) to a segment near the back of the spine—or dorsal region—called the **Dorsal Root Ganglion** (DRG), which houses their cell bodies and nuclei, where signals get processed before continuing to the region in the back of the spine known as **dorsal horn**.

It is at the junction with the dorsal horn where the sensory neurons have the option to connect at their segment, and/or several levels up or down. Once they enter the dorsal horn, their dendrites **synapse**—or chemically merge—with another type of neurons called **interneurons** or association neurons, a specialized multipolar neuron found only in the brain and spinal cord [18].

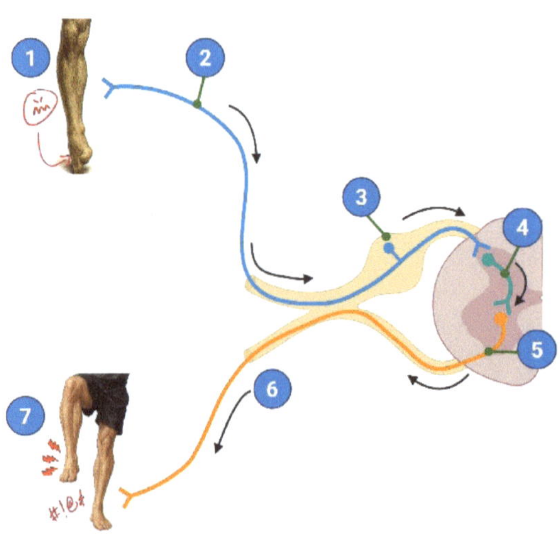

1. Injury and **injury detection**
2. Sensory neurons send signal to **DRG**
3. Signal processed at **DRG** and heading to **Dorsal Horn**
4. Signal relayed to **Interneuron** at **Dorsal Horn**
5. **Interneuron** relays **Protection Signal** to Motor Neurons
6. **Protection Signal** travels to periphery
7. **Protective Action** is executed

What makes these interneurons powerful is their integrative role as they synapse with the sensory neurons of multiple other structures in what is known as **convergence**, and also synapse with **motor neurons** connected to the front of the spine—or ventral region—where they will inhibit or stimulate different areas to create the appropriate protective response [19].

This protective loop is known as a **protective reflex arc**, **spinal reflex arc**, or just a **reflex**. It is instantaneous and beyond our conscious control [20]. The signal went from the ankle to the spine and instantly back to the leg for protection and balance without ever going to the brain. What will go to the brain is the pain signal.

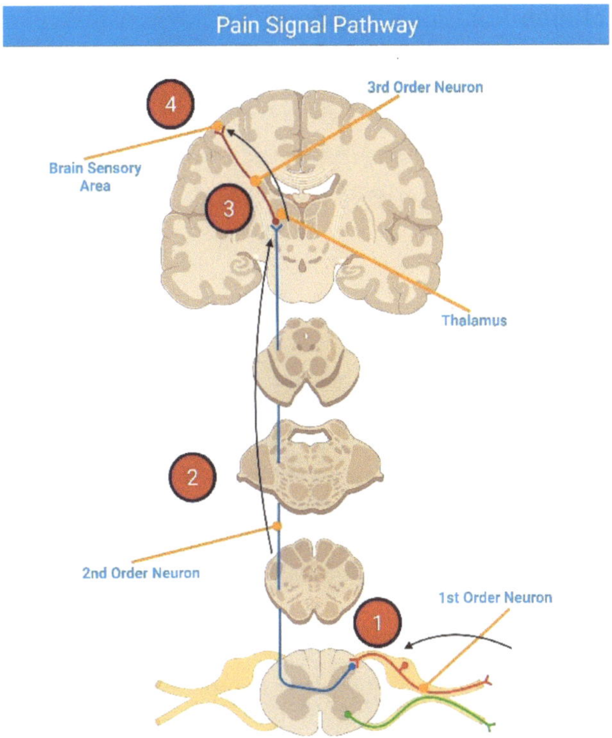

1) The pain signal arrives to the dorsal horn via the sensory neuron, the first order neuron in this sequence.

2) The signal then travels to the other side of the spine and then upward through the next neuron in the sensory upstream sequence, or second order neuron, which goes from the spine to the thalamus in the brain via the ascending tract, the equivalent of a spinal highway.

3) The signal then is relayed. to the thalamus, the proverbial gatekeeper, where it synapses with a third order neuron that travels to the sensory area of the brain.

4) At the sensory area the pain signal gets processed to produce a conscious response.

The manifestation and intensity of these responses is dependent on the extent of the injury and the perceptual state of the individual. Factors like shock, heightened emotional states, or other sources of endorphins, are known to momentarily dampen or even suppress pain signals [21].

What is undeniable is that the individual will eventually experience pain as the biochemistry around the injured ankle commences the healing process.

What Happens After

It is safe to assume that most of us are acquainted with the quirks of healing from an ankle sprain. The pain, discoloration, inflammation, rigidity, and weakness are impossible to ignore but also deter us from disrupting the healing process through conscious actions. These mechanisms may inconvenience us but they are actually beneficial.

This vast array of sensations and physical manifestations is orchestrated by multiple proinflammatory mediators, which are released in the onset of trauma, infection, allergic reactions, and even chronic stress. They include Norepinephrine, Substance P, Prostaglandins, Bradykinins [13], and protein-based molecules known as **cytokines** [22] [23] whose main role is to orchestrate tissue repair. Cytokines became mainstream vernacular with the advent of COVID-19 and the infamous cytokine storms that resulted from severe infections [24].

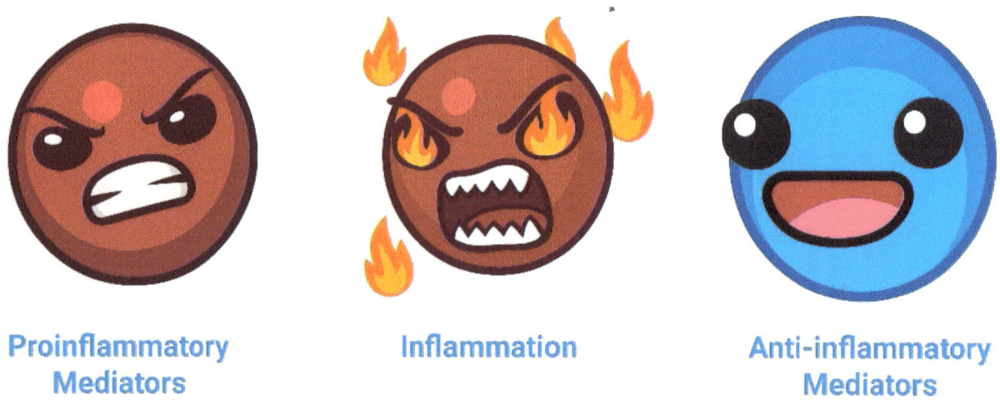

While the total number of cytokines is not known, a significant number of those involved in the perpetuation of pain and dysfunction are part of the interleukin subset of thirty-three cytokines [25], some of which are proinflammatory and some of which are anti-inflammatory. There are some non-interleukin cytokines also involved, which we'll review later on.

Inflammation is an essential component of the healing process and our bodies are designed to produce it and to drain it away, but this interaction can get disrupted by the entrapment of three cytokines identified as key players in the perpetuation of pain and dysfunction. They are **Tumor Necrosis Factor Alpha** (**TNF α**), **Interleukin 1β** (**IL 1β**), and **Interleukin 6** (IL 6) [13], which are produced in response to immune-system activation, trauma, and stress. In addition to perpetuating pain and dysfunction, these cytokines can potentially drive unfavorable changes in our physiology [26].

Under ideal circumstances, both proinflammatory and anti-inflammatory mediators work in harmony with our physiology to produce healing inflammation and to drain it when no longer necessary [27] [28].

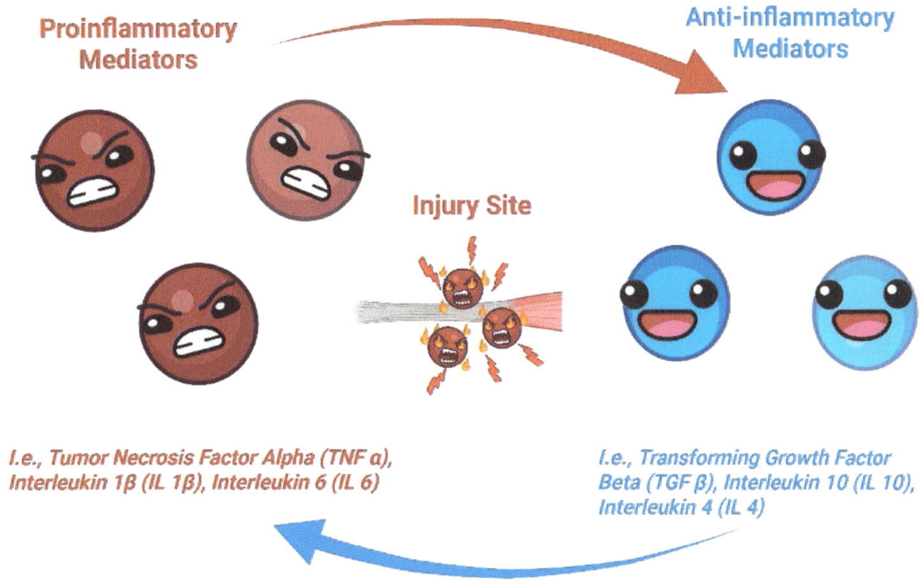

In our case of ankle injury, as ligaments, muscles, tendons, nerves, veins, arteries, and other structures heal to the point they can safely sustain mechanical loading, the inflammation needed for tissue repair is no longer necessary and gets washed away by **vascular perfusion**—the fluid-flow process through which the vascular structures bring nutrients and/or remove waste. This is when tight muscles let go and pain eases signaling that the injury has healed. It is what *should* happen after an injury.

But then again, we all know that this does *not* happen all the time.

Why What Should Have Happened Did Not

Few things are as frustrating as when pain and/or dysfunction linger long after an injury has physically healed, or when pain or dysfunction, including systemic conditions, appear without obvious causes. This is usually the result of protective reflex arcs—the same ones that engaged during the ankle sprain—getting stuck on a self-perpetuating loop, thus becoming *aberrant protective reflex arcs*.

Until recently, the factors leading to this abnormal response and the conditions arising from it were considered *idiopathic*—meaning of unknown cause—or even attributed to genetics, but the theorical driver presented in Brian's paper sheds light on the physiological interactions at their genesis.

In the case of the ankle injury, it's common to experience residual pain and dysfunction long after the bruises have faded and the ankle is back in commission. In many cases, one may also start experiencing pain and dysfunction in the knees, hips, or lower back areas. Though we tend to simplify the phenomena as musculoskeletal compensation, the inability of musculoskeletal methods to relieve them when the pain patterns get more complex [29] [30] makes us realize there's a component we're overlooking.

It is then that we turn our attention to trapped inflammation, where the main issue is figuring out where this inflammation is trapped. Conventional tests are not designed to recognize it, and if they look for it they'll look everywhere except where the inflammation is trapped. Which bring us to the question: *Where exactly is this inflammation trapped?*

We now know this, thanks to an important discovery that let us know that ...

Fascia is not Alone

I wonder if **Marvin Minsky** ever imagined the wonders his invention would reveal when he patented the confocal microscope in 1957 [31]. It has evolved to become confocal laser endomicroscopy, which can get real-time, high-resolution images of living tissue, thus opening new dimensions in medical procedures and research.

Interstitium Overview

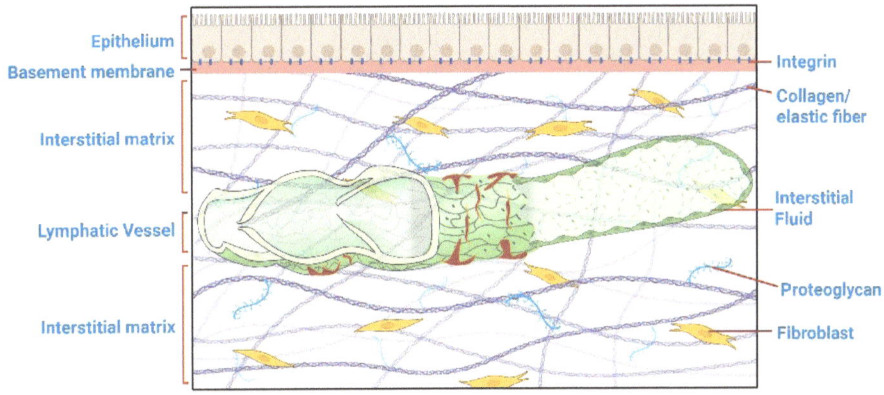

This is what made possible the histological breakthrough of 2018, where researchers identified pathways forming a complex network of collagen bundles filled with clear fluid that ***preceded the lymphatic networks*** [32]. Up to that point, these networks had only been seen as dense connective tissue, or even microtears.

Our bodies are designed to produce and remove inflammation. Under ideal circumstances, anti-inflammatory cytokines and normal interstitial fluid pressure drive efficient microvasculature drainage to clear proinflammatory mediators from the interstitium.

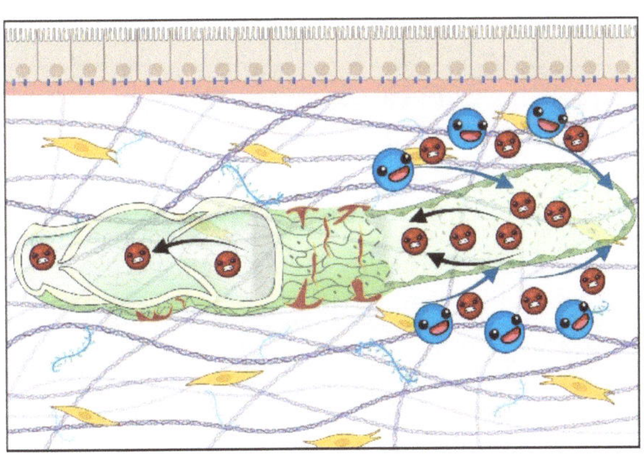

Injuries, infections, stress, etc., create mechanical and chemical blocks that disrupt microvasculature function, potentially trapping inflammation and proinflammatory mediators, and overpowering the anti-inflammatory response. The end result is Interstitial Inflammatory Stasis (IIS).

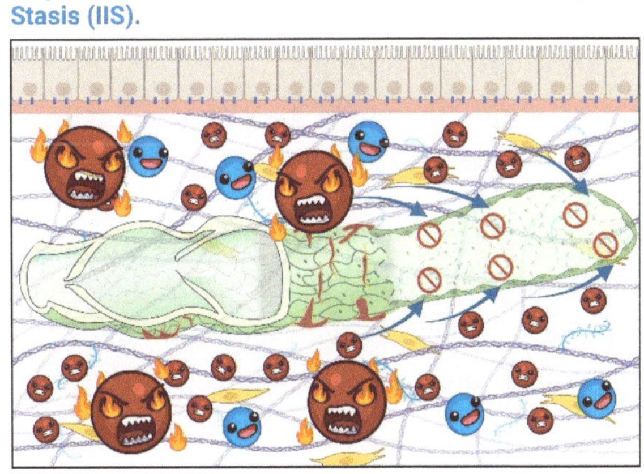

This complex collective of microscopic channels and vessels forming a microvascular system is known as the **interstitium.** Its anatomical distribution includes the dermis, vascular adventitia, submucosa of the viscera, bronchi, adipose tissue, and all fascial tissues, including musculoskeletal fascia. **This is where the inflammation and its proinflammatory mediators get trapped**, thus compromising our microvasculature, and tissue function and health.

The take-home message from this scientific article is clear: *Proper drainage is crucial for interstitial health, ergo, systemic health* [32]. Theoretically, the lymphatic system and vascular perfusion would clear all inflammation from the interstitium as the healing process comes to completion. However, the nature of the interstitium as a **pre-lymphatic layer** means that *any disruption to the microvasculature and vascular perfusion mechanisms could trap proinflammatory mediators.* This entrapment is known as **Interstitial Inflammatory Stasis (IIS).** It's from here that trapped inflammation travels to the spinal cord via the fascial sensory neurons, where it can generate self-perpetuating loops of pain and dysfunction. And, as previously mentioned, it can even change the nature of the surrounding tissues [13] [26].

None of us is impervious to the presence of inflammation, since it's essential for tissue health and repair. We all carry some and it's normal to live with different levels of asymptomatic inflammation. The tricky part is predicting whether the inflammation will get entrapped and become problematic. Because, for this to happen, *the proinflammatory markers have to accumulate to a level where they overpower the anti-inflammatory and inhibitory elements, thus crossing a threshold of tolerance* [33] [34].

The most salient evidence of trapped inflammation was the study conducted by Dr. Jay P Shah [14] [35]. He used a micro-dialysis needle to extract the interstitial fluid from an active trigger point on a symptomatic trapezius and compared it to the fluid in the asymptomatic side. He found that twenty-three different proinflammatory mediators—such as Substance P, Interleukin 6, Norepinephrine, etc.—were elevated on the affected side compared to the uninvolved side. This breakthrough corroborated the existence of trigger points, myofascial pain, and other systemic pains that until then were dismissed as psychological conditions because conventional bloodwork and imaging studies couldn't point to any established markers.

As to how inflammation travels to the spine, this can be understood by seeing nerves and neurons in a different light. The popular view equates them to one-way electric wires, where the orders come from the central nervous system. In reality, the neurons that make up the nerves are channels or tubes, where chemicals and signals are *sent to* **and** *received from* the spinal cord [36] [37]. As you will soon learn, this is how trapped inflammation travels to the spinal cord and how *the spinal cord itself can send inflammation to the periphery.*

Fascia ... Yes and No

But isn't the technique called *Fascial Counterstrain?* Why are we, then, diverting our attention away from fascia?

On the contrary! Allow me to illustrate.

There are moments when serendipities provide us with a much-needed new dimension of understanding. One such moment arrived in late 2019 as I worked on a new client. He was thrilled with his results but wanted to know what made Fascial Counterstrain different from other fascial modalities. He had previously seen another fascial therapist who claimed that his method was the same as Counterstrain.

"Your treatment is so different," he said. "But don't the two of you work on fascia?"

I think we all recognize a revelation. It arrives all at once and in a manner that defies linear time—a gift from a higher intelligence. I had a vision of connected networks and webs where energy traveled in an orderly fashion until it encountered a self-sustained area of congestion, where aberrant signals disrupted the harmony and continuum. I saw how powerful these congested areas were and how far their disruptions reached.

"Not really," I said. "I work with what affects fascia."

It was a crucial distinction that's helped me clarify Counterstrain from other fascial modalities. Back then I attributed it only to aberrant reflex arcs. Nowadays, the understanding of trapped inflammation makes this vision even more relatable. We are contemplating fascia from not just mechanistic views, but also from physiological and neural frames, which help us understand fascial microvasculature and its cellular health and behavior. Fascia in all its expressions will always be involved because it's surrounded by interstitium, and thus, susceptible to the effects of trapped inflammation, and that **source inflammation** is the target of our treatment.

Of Interneurons, Convergence, and Types of Inflammation

It is uncontestable that every one of our seven-trillion-plus nerve endings communicates with our brains. But this communication is not a direct pathway for most. Were this the case, as Brian constantly reminds us, our spinal cords would be the thickness of tree trunks [38]. Our bodies solve this conundrum via **neural convergence** at a structure that should now be familiar, the **interneuron**.

Recall that **interneurons,** or association neurons, serve an integrative role as they *synapse with the sensory neurons of multiple other structures* in what is known as **convergence**. One of my favorites illustrations of neural convergence is the one I learned from Brian Tuckey. We can think of the interneuron as a power strip, of the converging structures as appliances, of sensory neurons as their power cords, and of the plugs connecting to the outlets as synapses.

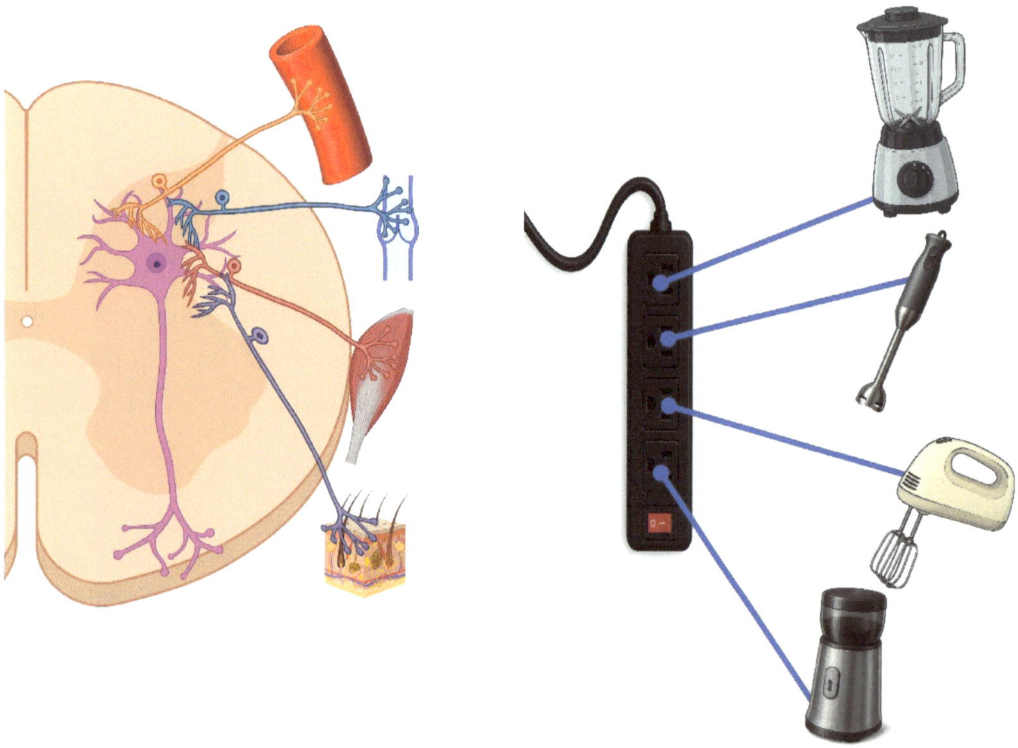

Different physiological structures converging at an interneuron via their sensory neurons, just like different appliances converge in a single power strip.

Just as a power strip allows to connect different low-power appliances to a power source without the need of multiple dedicated outlets, the interneurons allow different physiological structures to communicate with the spine without the bulk of dedicated connections. And this is as far as I'll go with this analogy. Any further, and we'll run into the risk of oversimplification.

Neural convergence—as it relates to FCS—is far more interactive with our physiology and internal environment. A brief look of the most salient components allows us to contemplate why understanding this concept is crucial in FCS mastery.

Neural Convergence Example

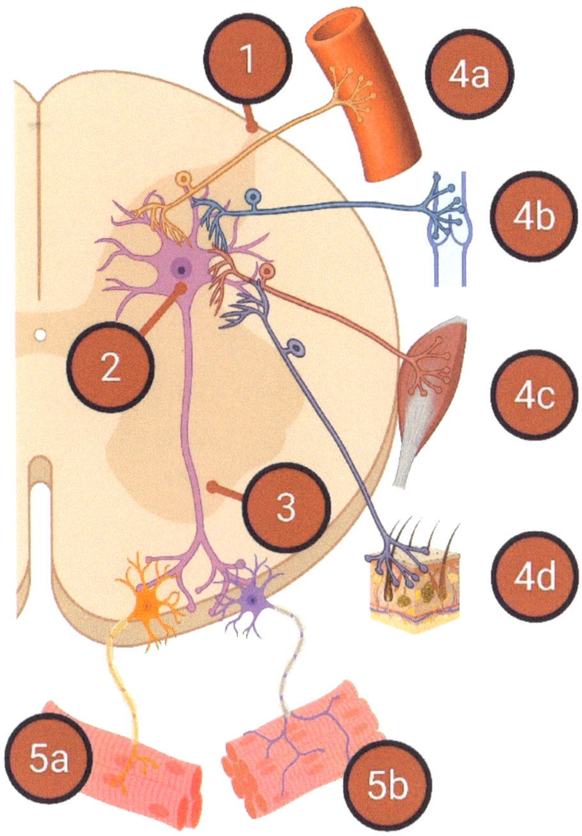

1) Dorsal Horn – Back of the spinal cord region, where the sensory neurons enter to access the deeper spinal structures.

2) Interneuron – Multipolar neuron found only in the spinal cord and brain. This is where the sensory neurons from different structures converge.

3) Ventral Horn – Front of spinal cord region, where interneurons relay their message to synapsing motor neurons.

4) Convergence – Of different fascial expressions at the same interneuron via their sensory neurons, including 4a) arterial fascia, 4b) venous fascia, 4c) myofascia, and 4d) skin fascia.

5) Motor Neuron Synapses – With the interneuron at the ventral horn to produce either 5a) motor neuron activation or 5b) motor neuron inhibition.

Another factor that makes neural convergence so influential is that interneurons also synapse with **motor neurons** connected to the front of the spine—or ventral region—where they inhibit or stimulate different musculoskeletal or smooth muscle (vasculature and organs) areas to create the appropriate protective response.

Now that we understand the components of neural convergence, we can explore how inflammation travels from the affected structure to the interneuron, where it'll create the cascade of responses typical of pain and dysfunction.

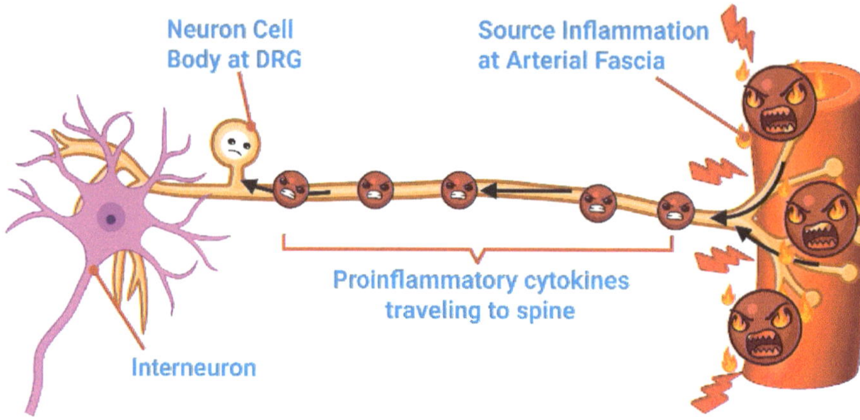

Recall that neurons are tubes and that all fascial expressions are rich in type III and IV pain-sensing neurons, or nociceptors. Once an injured or affected structure starts producing inflammation, it will send this source inflammation toward the spine via these sensory neurons, where it will first affect their bodies and nuclei at the *Dorsal Root Ganglion* (DRG) [38].

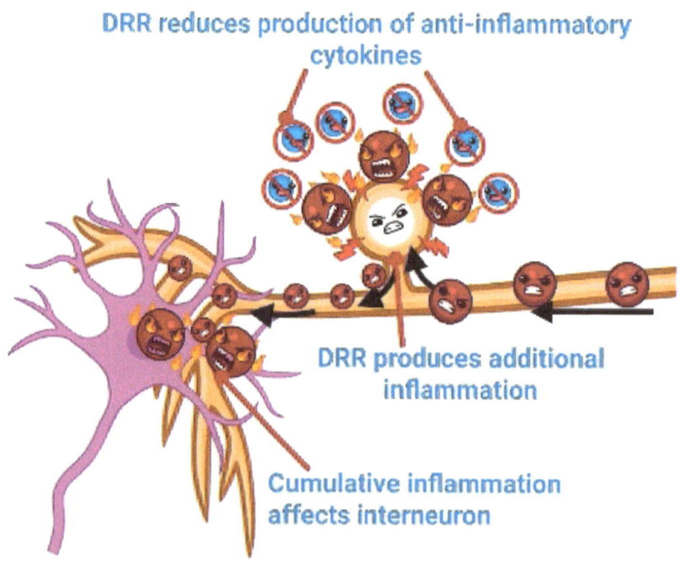

In the case of Type III and IV nociceptors connected to the fascial networks, the entire neuron gets sensitized by two factors. First, the neuronal cell bodies at the DRG react to the presence of inflammation by increasing their reactivity [23]. And second, the presence of inflammatory mediators at the neuronal body elicits the *Dorsal Root Reflex* (DRR) [39], which combined with the increased reactivity, essentially makes the entire neuron more likely to fire to minor stimuli. The DRR will also drive the affected neuronal body to produce additional proinflammatory cytokines, and to reduce the production of anti-inflammatory mediators [40].

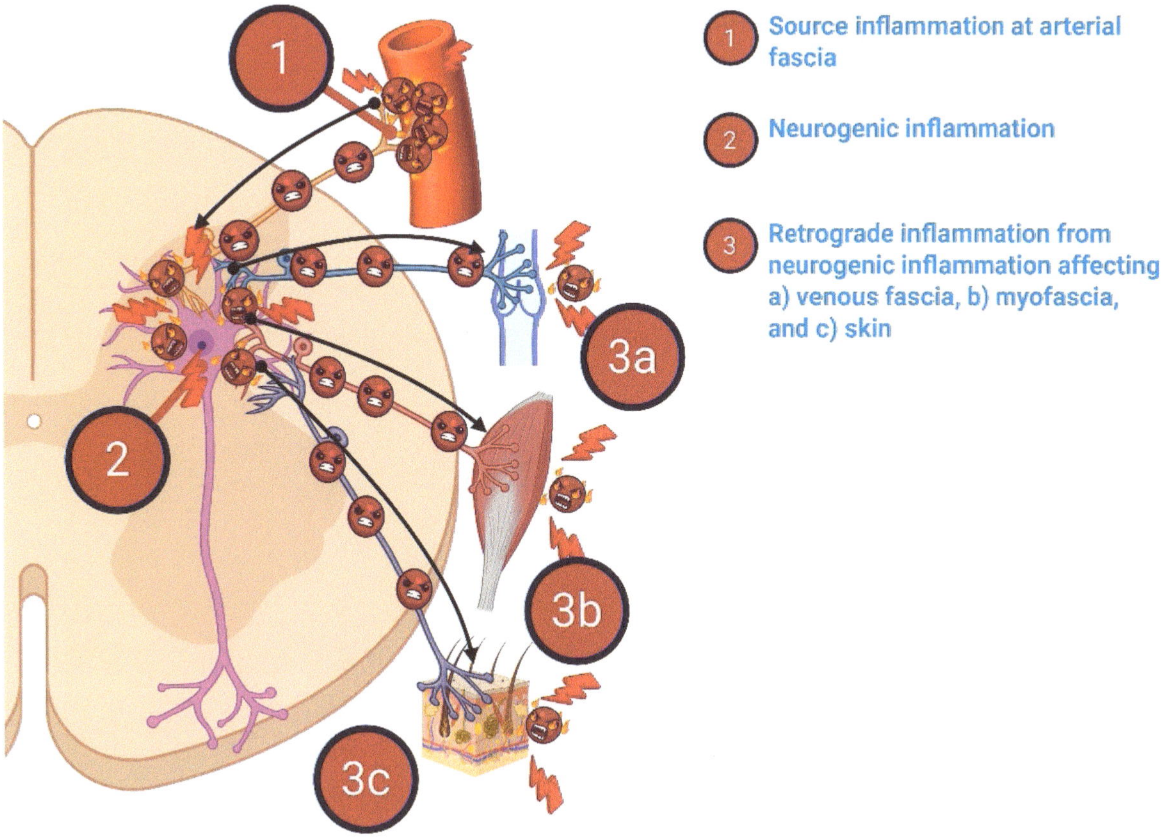

After affecting the DRG, the inflammation continues to the dorsal horn of the spine, where the sensory neuron synapses with an interneuron. It then inflames the synapsing interneuron and *all* its convergent neurons, producing a type of inflammation known as **Neurogenic Inflammation** [41]. This neurogenic inflammation travels then through the affected neurons in the convergence in a *retrograde* direction to their connected structures in the periphery, where it collects as **Retrograde Inflammation** and creates other loops of aberrant reflex arcs.

Depending on their location, these loops will affect muscle guarding reflexes, heart rate, blood pressure, organ function, or a combination of them [13].

But there's a particularly disruptive type of inflammation: when the source inflammation originates in the glial cells of the CNS (astrocytes, microglia, oligodendrocytes, etc., found only in the brain and spine) rather than the periphery. Events such as concussions, whiplashes, meningitis, subdural empyema, spinal surgeries, or chronic stress affect the central nervous system directly.

Neuroinflammation Drivers

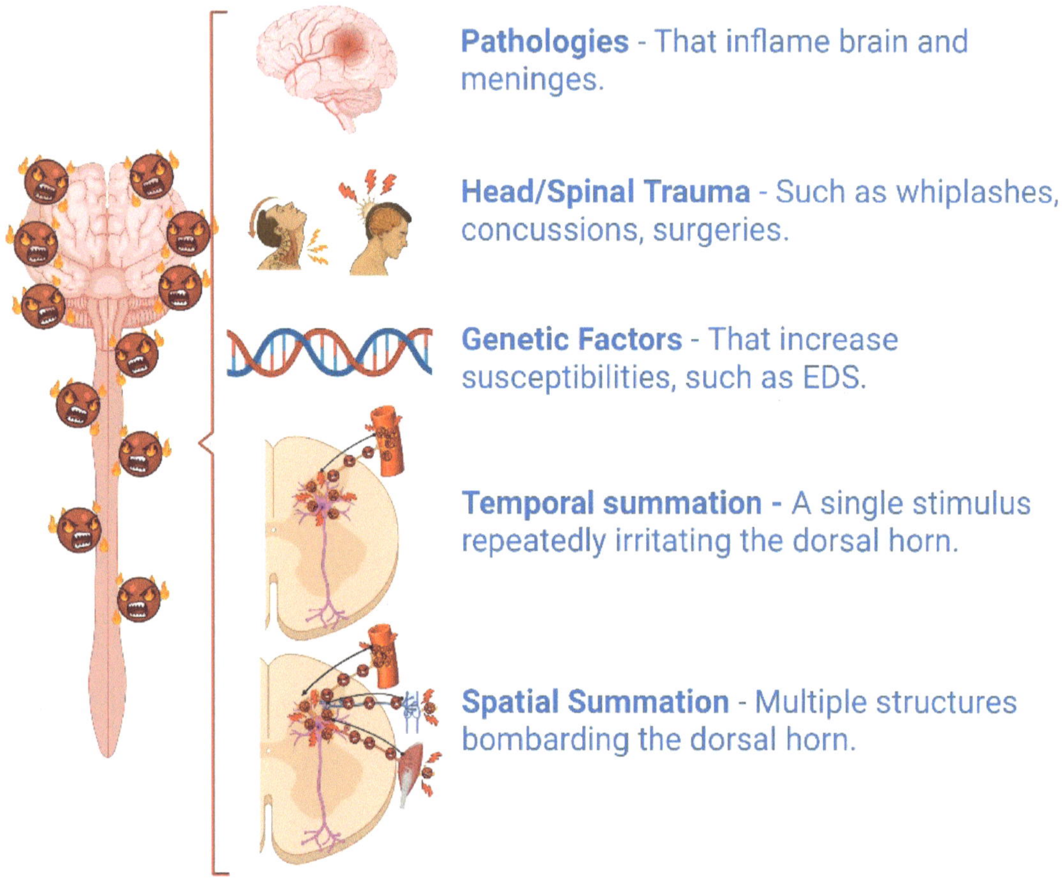

Glial cells can also get inflamed when the loops of peripheral inflammation are so high that they overwhelm the CNS. This bombardment can be driven by *temporal summation*, which is a single stimulus repeatedly irritating the dorsal horn; or *spatial summation*, which is multiple structures affecting the dorsal horn.

The resulting inflammation in the CNS—whether from the glial cells or from peripheral bombardment—is known as **Neuroinflammation** [42] which drives the **Central Sensitization** [43] that affects large segments of the body and/or entire organ systems.

Neuroinflammation is also linked to the transition from acute pain to chronic pain, and central sensitization is theorized to increase resistance to opioids by altering neuronal function [44]. Neural convergence is powerful and can explain a multitude of interacting phenomena, including one the most recognized assessment elements for the therapist and the client: *tender points*.

Neural Convergence and Tender Points

The use of tender points is not unique to Counterstrain. You may be familiar with the more popular *trigger point* moniker and you may have experienced a form of therapy that targets them.

It should be noted that the consensus on trigger points and tender points sharing commonalities but not being the same entity is changing. Both manifest locally and in distant locations, both can identified as hyperirritable nodules in a taut band of skeletal muscle, or as nodules at the skin level in bones, ligaments, tendons, bursae, and fat pads. Though trigger points are more characteristic of myofascial pain and tender points are more characteristic of fibromyalgia, they have been found to share a common pathophysiology [26].

What's crucial to remember is that in Fascial Counterstrain **we *do not* treat the tender points, but rather, their symptom-driving structures**, which are the structures harboring the source inflammation.

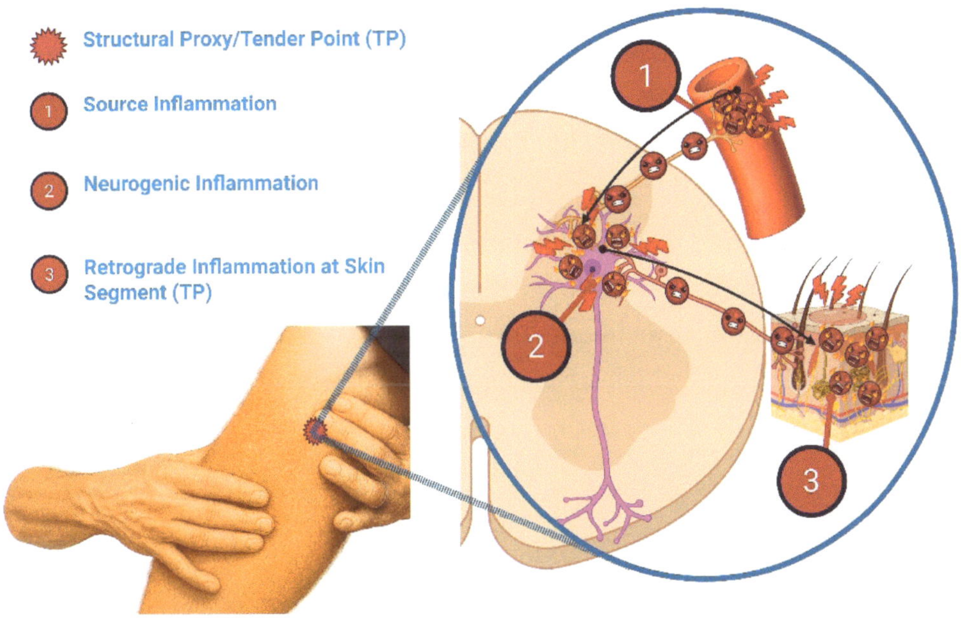

As recently stated, what affects one neuron in a convergence affects all the neurons in that convergence. It turns out that all deep spinal neurons also converge in a segment of the skin. Thus, any inflammation affecting that convergence will also inflame that segment of the skin. This small area of retrograde inflammation is the tender point, and since it's the proxy of the target structure harboring the source inflammation, it can be used to monitor treatment.

The palpatory sensations at the tender point let us know whether our technique is optimal, insufficient, or excessive. These sensations also let us know when treatment is approaching peak, when it's concluded, or not working at all. In essence, by draining the trapped source inflammation from our target structure, we're also draining the inflammation from all the converging structures including the skin [38].

One does not have to experience pain to have tender points. It is common to find them in asymptomatic areas during treatment, much to the surprise of the client who didn't know they existed. These tender points are considered *subthreshold* or *latent*, meaning their inflammation hasn't crossed the threshold. But that doesn't make them innocuous. As they continue irritating the dorsal horn via *temporal summation* and/or or *spatial summation*, they sensitize the spine, thus making us more susceptible to react to a minor stimulus.

Neural Convergence and Muscle Tightness

Who has not experienced the neck, shoulder, or hip knots and tightness we love to pound or subjugate to forceful stretches? It seems obvious to give them the attention because they are the ones making the noise, but while those knotty tight muscles are reliable indicators of pain and dysfunction, they are not the culprit [45].

To understand how IIS produces palpable and measurable muscular changes, we must remember that the source inflammation travels to the dorsal horn of the spine—the sensory area—where it affects all neurons converging in an interneuron. Synapsing with the interneuron on the opposite end, we find the motor neurons, which are in charge of voluntary and involuntary movement, and exit the spine from the ventral (front) horn.

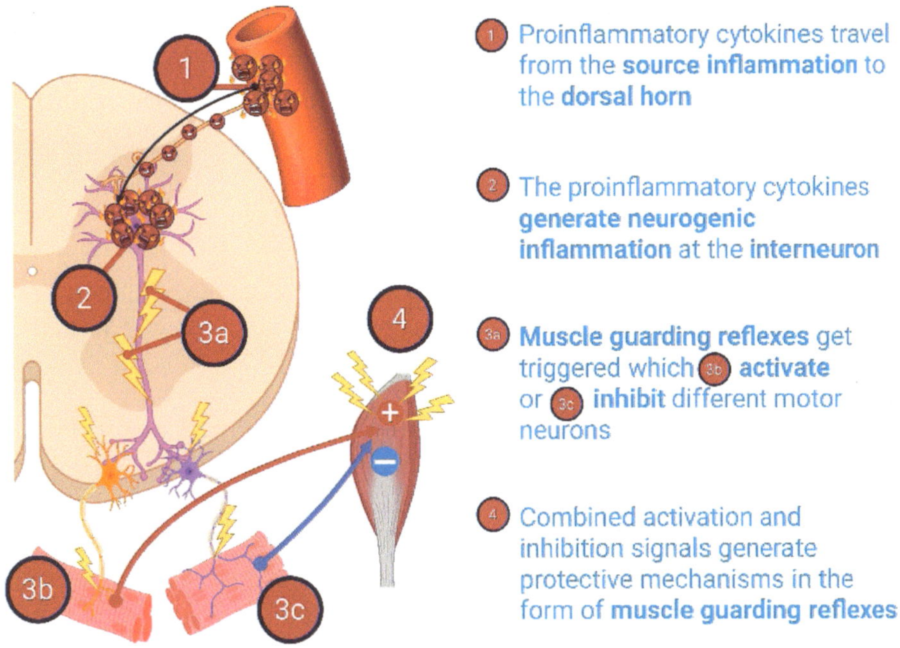

The activation of these motor neurons from this inflammation creates *muscle guarding reflexes*, which means the muscles go into a protective contracted state. The involuntary contraction is theorized to be attempts by the body to decompress the affected area [13] [38] and to discourage us from exacerbating the condition through our physical actions. Because this is a reflexive response, the muscular tightness will remain—even at rest—until the source inflammation dissipates.

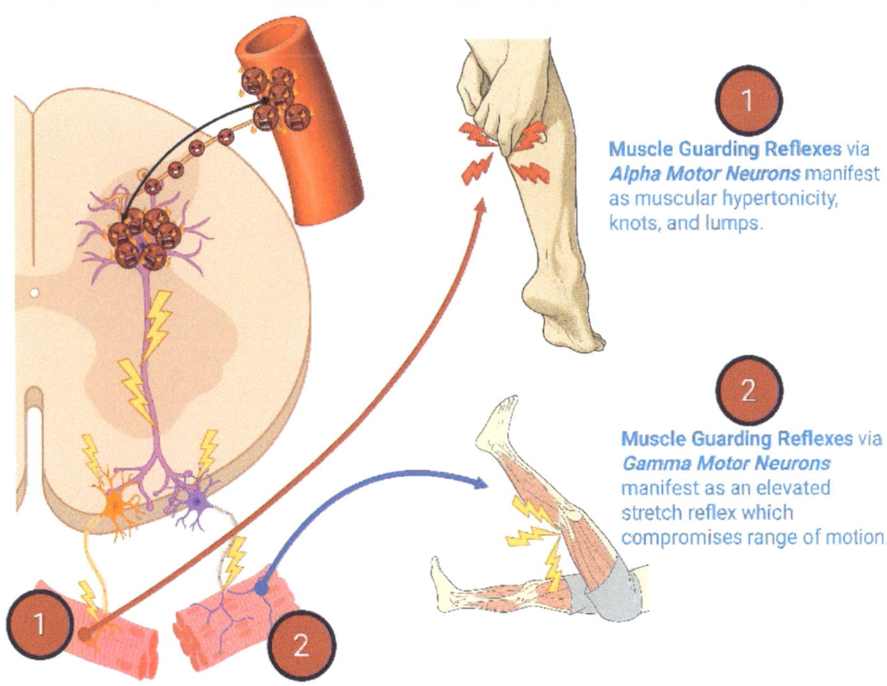

The nature of this muscle guarding reflex will vary depending on which motor neurons are affected [46]. Activation of the **alpha motor neurons** produces the all-too-familiar hypertonicity and muscular lumps we eagerly poke and compress, whereas activation of the **gamma motor neurons** produces an elevated stretch reflex, which compromises range of motion. Think of tight hamstrings that, while not rigid at rest, still fail to achieve a functional range of motion.

The proficient therapist will notice the muscular rigidity and/or reduced range of motion but won't try to fix them directly. Instead, the attention will be directed to finding the source inflammation because draining it will restore tissue health and motion without direct intervention.

Pain ... but Which One?

Barring exogenous substances or high-emotion events that produce high levels of inhibitory elements [21], the sensation we know as pain is experienced immediately upon injury. Since we're dealing with the aftermath that perpetuates pain and dysfunction, we'll limit the topic to what we address in Fascial Counterstrain: *Interstitial Inflammatory Stasis* (IIS).

We acknowledge the client's perceived pain, but we also acknowledge that—because of IIS and neural convergence—all pains are different, and thus, have to be approached differently. There are three expressions of pain we commonly find and they're determined by the location of the trapped inflammation

Hyperalgesia. The most unmistakable sign of inflammatory stasis in a structure. These are localized areas of exaggerated sensitivity to touch, may even be the original areas of injury [47], and—as it pertains to Counterstrain—have the greatest effect on other areas because they harbor the primary or **source inflammation**. Think of the ankle-sprain example. In that specific case, the source inflammation is at the site of injury and draining it produces the most benefits.

All neurogenic inflammation is a reaction to this source inflammation bombarding the dorsal horn. This neurogenic inflammation will then be sent in a retrograde direction to all the neurons in a convergence and collect as retrograde inflammation in their structures. The pain and dysfunction experienced in these areas of retrograde inflammation is known as secondary hyperalgesia.

Secondary Hyperalgesia. Whereas hyperalgesia is an expression of the source inflammation, *secondary hyperalgesia* is an expression of the retrograde inflammation. Secondary hyperalgesia creates confusion as it produces pain and dysfunction on uninjured tissues and won't respond to direct treatment [48]. All tender points are expressions of secondary hyperalgesia [26] even if derived from the source inflammation. The difference is that draining the tender point from the source inflammation will produce an immediate therapeutic response, whereas the tender points generated by retrograde inflammation won't respond to treatment.

Let's revisit our ankle sprain, and let's suppose it's been over a year since the incident. The pain persists, and it's spread to the knee, hip, and low back. Assessment shows that the ankle has no remarkable swelling, but it has a distinctive tender point indicating that the tunica adventitia of a vascular structure is harboring the source inflammation. While the knee, hip, and low back are also affected, the assessment indicates they're only a byproduct of the source inflammation from the ankle. Without getting too elaborate, draining the source inflammation from the ankle also drains the retrograde inflammation affecting the knee, hip, and low back.

Allodynia. Can be summarized as an extreme sensitivity to pain, and along with sensory issues and organ dysfunctions, the likely results of central sensitization—when the source inflammation is neuroinflammation from the CNS. Allodynia can be so pronounced that we experience pain from an otherwise benign stimulus, such as the sensation from the clothes we're wearing or from a gentle hug [43]. It is also common to experience significant pain and dysfunction but lack tender points.

As a result, the client may find conventional treatment uncomfortable and relief unpredictable. While there are simpler cases of central sensitization that can be addressed by pretty much anyone, a significant number requires an advanced Counterstrain Therapist capable of accessing and recognizing the intricacies of a sensitized CNS. It is not until this source neuroinflammation is drained that the client starts noticing changes and experiencing relief.

But there's another aspect of this inflammatory stasis besides the pain, dysfunction, and tightness. IIS has a latent side-effect that potentially perpetuates its presence and compromises cellular health [13].

Trapped Inflammation and Our Physiology

Heightened sensitivity, tissue degeneration, and/or organ issues are common in clients dealing with different systemic conditions, not just chronic pain. This is where the IIS hypothesis provides us with novel perspectives in possible mechanisms.

It is important to understand how trapped inflammation is at the genesis of the evident symptomology, but it's also important to understand how this IIS alters our physiology and, in so doing, perpetuates its presence and creates unfavorable changes.

Increased Nerve Sensitivity

Pain, swelling, and burning as a result of a recent injury—that's how inflammation is popularly viewed. Rarely is it even considered in chronic pain, or in how reactive to a minor stimulus an area becomes. *How can it be inflammation when it happened a long time ago?*

Let's review some key details:

- All forms of fascia are surrounded by interstitium.
- It's in the interstitium where the source inflammation gets trapped.
- Type III and IV nociceptors are the most abundant sensory neurons in all forms of fascia.
- The source inflammation affecting the interstitium also affects its fascia and nociceptors.
- Nociceptors are neurons, ergo, tubes or channels, the perfect highway for the inflammatory mediators to travel from the source inflammation to the spine.

As previously mentioned, the inflammation will arrive first to the neuron body/nucleus at the Dorsal Root Ganglia (DRG), thus activating the *Dorsal Root Reflex* (DRR) [39] which combined with the increased reactivity of the affected neuron reduces the level of stimulus needed to make it fire. Though the injury may have happened in the past, the presence of IIS continues sensitizing the nerve, making it more likely to react to what would be considered mundane activities.

Cessation of the Lymphatic Pumps

Our lymphatic system increases its lymphangion activity (*more on lymphangions later*) in the presence of many inflammatory mediators [49]. However, this intrinsic, homeostatic, clearing system sometimes falls short leading to excess inflammation and disease [13].

Recent research has shown us that this could be attributed to the three previously mentioned proinflammatory cytokines. It's been observed during acute inflammatory events that **Tumor Necrosis Factor Alpha (TNF α)**, **Interleukin 1β (IL 1β)**, and **Interleukin 6 (IL 6)** can disable the local lymphatic pumps [50]. This is hypothesized to be a defense mechanism to avoid spreading infection and/or inflammation beyond the affected areas. Effective as this defensive mechanism is, it also has the potential to create IIS because the research has also shown that while the **systemic lymphatic pump** eventually recovers, the **local lymphatic pump** may remain disabled [13].

A disabled local lymphatic pump means trapped inflammation, which in turn is the catalyst for other unfavorable physiological changes.

Scarring and Fibrosis

When it comes to bone spurs, fibrosis, or keloid scarring, the consensus is to blame genetics or aging. Rarely does one think of trapped inflammation as a possible driver. And yet, thanks to Brian Tuckey connecting the dots, we can now see how IIS is at the genesis of many of these dysfunctions.

We mentioned how **Tumor Necrosis Factor Alpha** (**TNF α**), **Interleukin 1β** (**IL 1β**), and **Interleukin 6** (**IL 6**) have the ability to disable the local lymphatic pumps It should be also mentioned that when the aforementioned cytokines are present for extended periods, they drive the production of **Transforming Growth Factor Beta One** (**TGF β1**). This powerful cytokine has two significant effects:

1. **It Causes Fascial Contraction.** When the fibroblasts—the core cells of fascial structures—are exposed to **TGF β1** they react by contracting. This further prolongs inflammatory entrapment and creates a state of hypoxia from fascial compression in the microvasculature of the involved structures and/or organ systems [13]. The issue is compounded by the inevitable muscle guarding reflexes that further compress the microvascular networks [51].
2. **It Changes Fibroblasts into Myofibroblasts.** Before one vilifies myofibroblasts, keep in mind that, though rare, this contractile cell occurs naturally in many structures of our bodies [52]. Also, the transformation of fibroblasts into myofibroblasts is a normal part of wound healing and repair [53]. It becomes problematic when the presence of **IL 1β**, **IL 6**, and **TGF β1** drive this change in an inflammatory entrapment state.

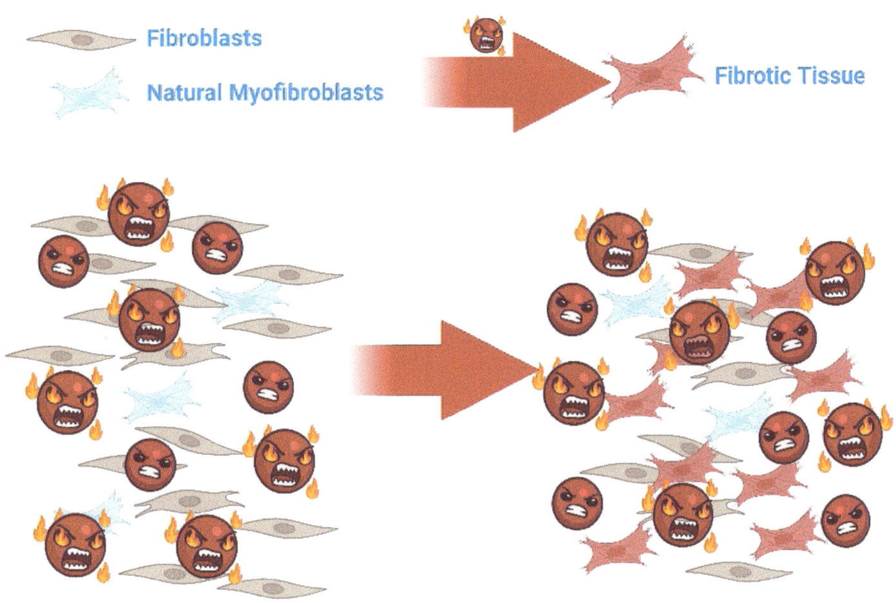

Compounding to this problem, all these myofibroblasts secrete additional **IL 1β**, **IL 6** and **TGF β1** among other cytokines, thereby increasing mechanical fascial contraction and the rate of unfavorable cellular transformation. That means that under the prolonged presence of trapped inflammation, healthy tissue starts turning into fibrotic, or scar, tissue [54], and not just in our musculoskeletal structures but also in organs and vasculature.

As if that were not enough, this IIS also affects the sympathetic division of the autonomic nervous system, which has the potential to affect perceptual states and entire organ systems.

Sympathetic Activation

Though we had mentioned that fascia and interstitium surround every structure in our bodies, we had limited our illustrations to the orthopedic realm of an ankle sprain. We can now add the remaining layer, which is the effects of IIS on the sympathetic division of the autonomic nervous system.

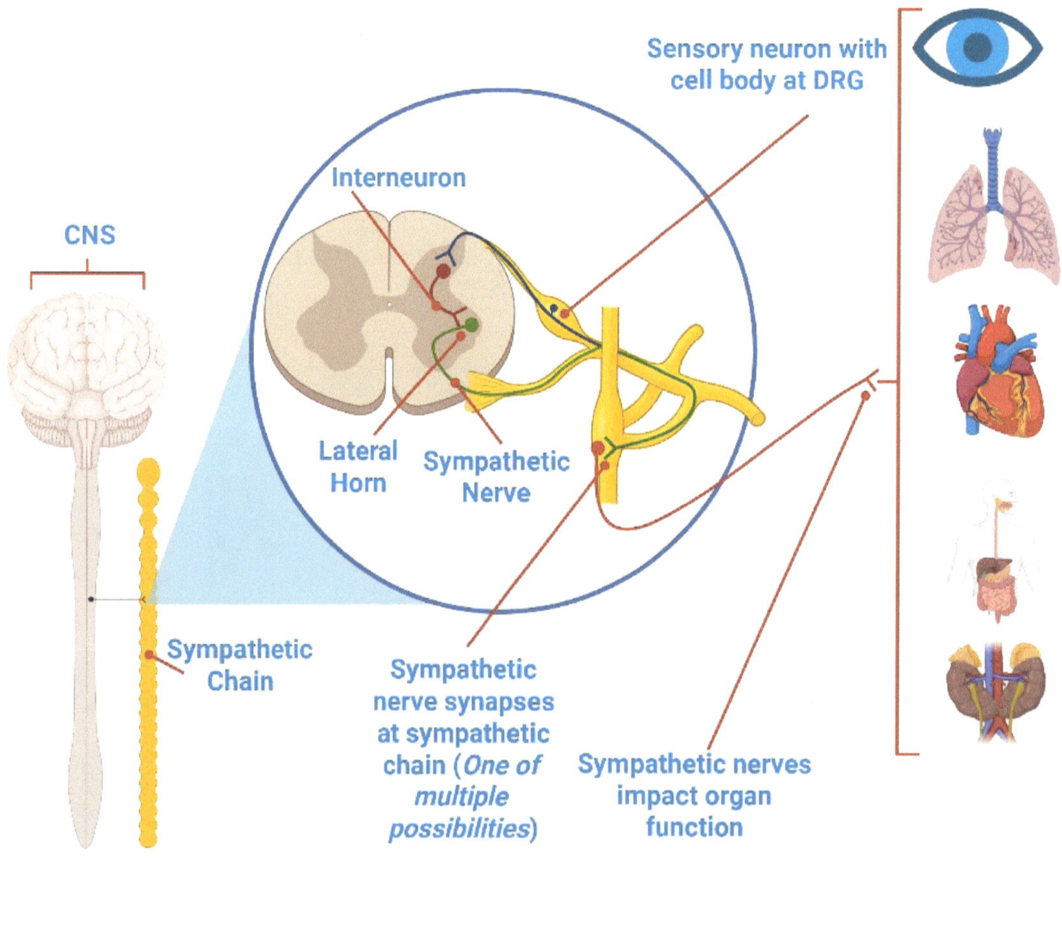

We know of the dorsal horn of the spine, where the sensory nerves enter to relay their message. We also know of the ventral horn of the spine, where the motor neurons come out to execute movement. And we also know of the interneuron, responsible for integrating the signals between the dorsal and ventral horns of the spine via their synapses.

But there's one more structure in the spine. And though it's only present from the very first segment of the thoracic spine (T1) to the second segment of the lumbar spine (L2), it connects with other structures to power the entire body [55].

It is the **lateral horn of the spine** which houses the neuronal cell bodies of the sympathetic nervous system which converge with nociceptors from the periphery, organs, as well as motor neurons via interneurons. This has important implications in the presence of IIS:

- **When the inflammatory insult comes from the periphery** (skin, muscles, joints, etc.,) the ensuing *somato-sympathetic reflexes* affect not only musculoskeletal structures, but also functions such as blood pressure, and organ systems.
- **When the inflammatory insult comes from the organs,** the ensuing *visceral-sympathetic reflexes* affect physiological functions, organs, and their peripheral muscle guarding reflexes [13]. Think of people enduring significant flank and back pain as they pass kidney stones.

Activation of the aforementioned reflexes will signal the release of epinephrine, which produces vasoconstriction [56] and may reduce local muscular blood flow by up to 25%, which the body's natural vasodilation responses cannot seem to overcome. These reflexes can also drive vasoconstriction of spinal arteries and veins, which could be at the genesis of many idiopathic conditions as well as degenerative disc or joint disease [13].

Activation of the sympathetic division from IIS has the potential to makes us more susceptible to other types of pain inputs [21] and alters our perceptual/mental health since this division is in charge of the proverbial *fight or flight* response. This can further disrupt blood-flow mechanics [57] and can also disrupt organ health [58].

Understanding and addressing all those interactions is what makes Fascial Counterstrain so powerful. It's what allows us to treat conditions that are not typical of conventional manual therapy. At this point, the core principle of the direction of ease should start making more sense, so it's time to see it with a new set of eyes.

The Direction of Ease Revisited

We had mentioned that the direction of ease is a direction of decompression that allows the body to drain the trapped inflammation [14]. It should now be clear that there's nothing random or phantasmal about it. Instead, we can appreciate how FCS turns all these complex interactions into a simple, elegant, gentle, and effective technique.

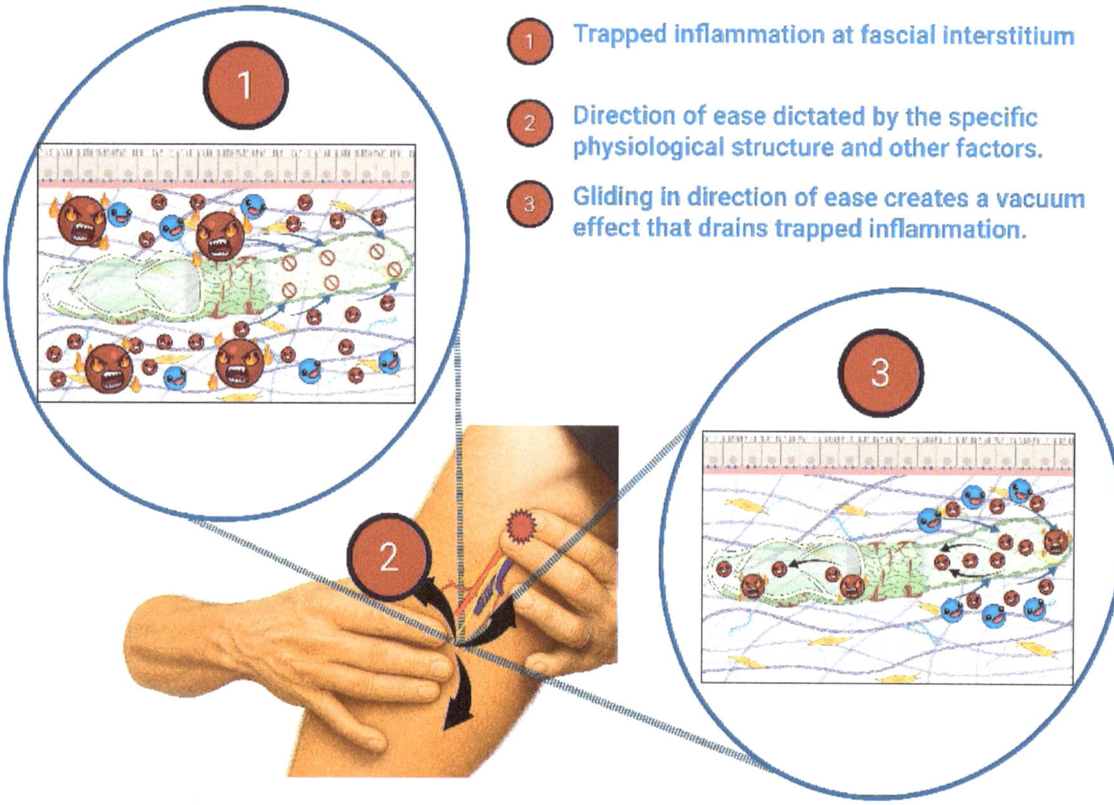

Let's recall that IIS creates mechanical blocks through reflexive fascial contraction and muscle guarding reflexes. It's the physical expressions of those reflexes that lead us to the source inflammation and its proxy tender point. We do *not* treat the tender point because it's only an expression of retrograde inflammation, but we use it to confirm the involved structure and to monitor treatment progress.

What we treat is the structure harboring the source inflammation by applying gentle pressure to engage its fascial structures, and then follow its direction of ease. This direction of ease is determined by the physiological characteristics of the involved structure. Treatments for arteries, nerves, and veins may start in the same area but have different directions of ease. The direction of ease is also affected by the presence of scarring, fibrosis, or anatomical variations.

The increased interstitial pressure created by the surplus fluids from IIS is one of the factors that stops inflammation and proinflammatory mediators from accessing the lymphatic channels [59]. The direction of ease takes advantage of this elevated pressure and the mechanical tension from the anchoring filaments at the lymphatic channels. It creates a vacuum effect that extracts all the surplus elements back to circulation for elimination.

With the source inflammation removed, the noxious bombardment affecting the DRG and interneuron stops and the protective reflexes are shut off. This allows our natural perfusion mechanisms to resume so that any leftover retrograde inflammation in converging structures can be drained without interference.

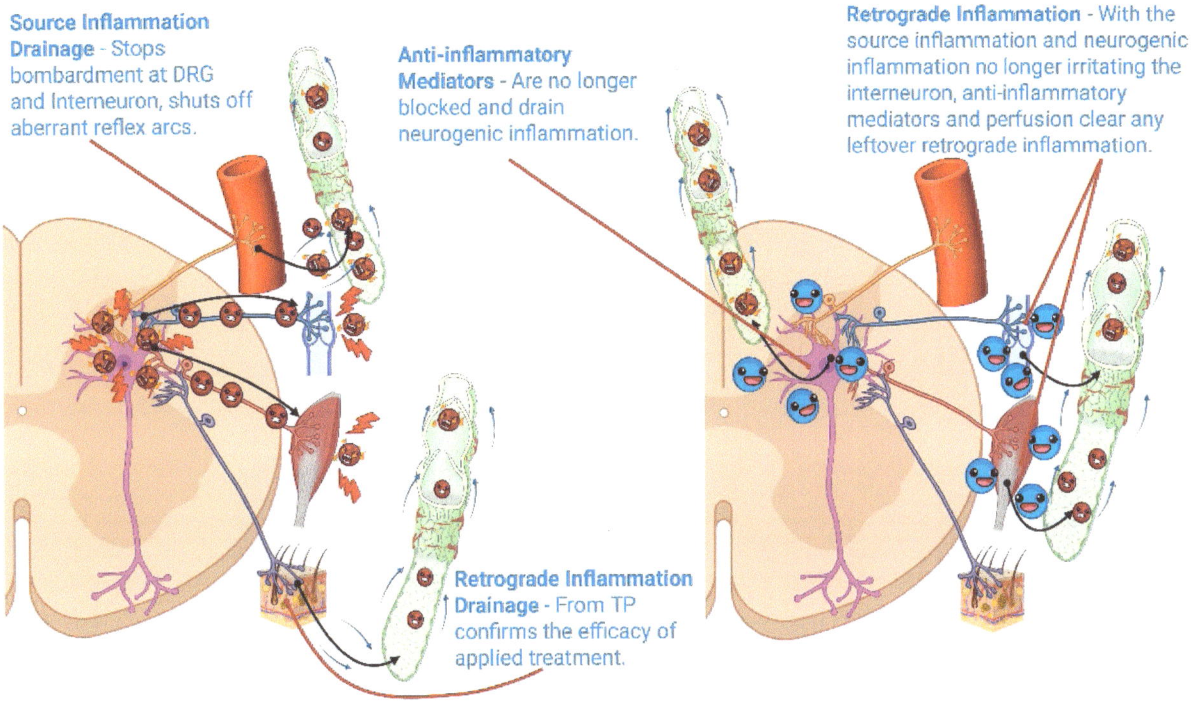

Provided that no other injurious or inflammatory insults are added, the anti-inflammatory mediators can handle any leftover neurogenic and retrograde inflammation on their own. That's why we encourage clients to fully rest and relax for at least two days after a session.

Now that the essence of principles dictating the mechanics of treatment are no longer a mystery, we can explore what Counterstrain means to the client and how the therapist arrives at the key areas of dysfunction.

THE COUNTERSTRAIN EXPERIENCE

"The line between the creative and the absurd is so thin, it often gets recklessly crossed."

COACH IZZY

Our imagination is the birthplace of creativity. When fueled by curiosity, research, and objective observation, it creates solutions to the most complex problems. Absent any of those qualities, it reinforces biases and fabricates misconceptions with enviable confidence.

There are two misconceptions I encounter frequently, and the first one involves the understanding of our modality. Fascial Counterstrain (FCS) is a fairly new field and as such, not easily relatable to those who have yet to experience it. Also, its indirect nature makes it hard to compare, and the more one tries to do so, the more confusion one creates. For starters, because the term *Fascial* is part of the name, many presume to understand it without having explored it.

The amount of misinformation about fascia in popular online content fuels much of the conceptual distortions. This content opens innocuously by reminding us that fascia is the largest living tissue in our bodies, that it connects us from the outside in, from the inside out, from head to toe and vice versa. No arguments there.

But then, despite all the evidence, it reduces fascia to a singular expression and focuses only on myofascia and myofascial treatment. Not surprisingly, those not acquainted with our field are certain that Counterstrain is yet another form of myofascial manipulation. Imagine their shock when they learn that while myofascia is real and treatable, it's not the Holy Grail of causality, nor the sole driver of pain and dysfunction, and there are multiple fascial expressions that the popular articles ignore or dismiss.

The second aspect is one that's been propagated by those claiming that their techniques are the only ones treating the root of the problem.

You have probably noticed that I continuously refer to the *source inflammation*—a term that I learned from Brian Tuckey—as the driver of the aberrant protective reflex arcs, which in turn manifest as pains, local dysfunctions, or systemic dysfunctions. When I talk about the mechanics of FCS, the term I use is *source inflammation* not *root of the problem*. The topic of the root of the problem is a multilayered theme I have to clarify to clients who believe, or want to be certain, that I target the root of the problem— the proverbial magical key to effortless healing. But is there really such a thing?

The Root of the Problem?

Finding the root of the problem is the Philosophers' Stone of medicine, where professionals from all modalities strive to find the factor that will bring magical, quick, and definite relief, and also serve as a fail-proof packageable template. Despite the tiffs among the experts who contradicted each other with their claims, the concept caught my attention early in my career.

But the more I studied the expert claims, the more clarity eluded me. Take, for instance, the concept of muscular imbalances as the root of the problem, never mind that the majority of muscular actions are unconscious and not necessarily indicative of a pathology [11]. Or pointing *fascial tightness* as the root of the problem and prescribing obsessive fascia stretching, never mind that fascia cannot be elongated [60] [61] and actually doing so would disrupt tissue length-tension relationships and impact inherent biomechanics. Let's not forget that fascia can remain pathologically contracted in the presence of trapped inflammation, which can give the illusion of tightness that no amount of stretching will ever fix.

Then again, irrespective of the claims, people were finding relief with these experts. *Who was I to question them?* Maybe there truly was a root of the problem.

Realizations and Reluctance

My first two years in Counterstrain were a roller coaster of revelations, learning, relearning, and unlearning. Much of what I had embraced as infallible crumbled—except for my obsession with the root of the problem. And I believed that Counterstrain was the only one that could find it. How could I not when the process guided me swiftly and accurately to the affected area?

However, as my cases grew in complexity, I had difficulty getting to *the root of the problem* consistently. These cases had erratic dysfunctions that would not respond to treatment. In many instances, treating the correct structures would unleash a barrage of new pain in different systems. Several of my experienced colleagues were also running into the same issues.

Fortunately, Brian Tuckey was already miles ahead in his research and advancing the field. As I acquired the new knowledge and skills, and I learned from Brian about the source inflammation and what creates it, I realized that draining it was only a step of the process and that the root of the problem was not singular and definite as popularly portrayed.

In my experience, Counterstrain goes to the source inflammation, which is the root of aberrant reflex arcs but not necessarily the root of the problem. *It is the events or circumstances that produce inflammation that I consider to be the root of the problem*, which can be the result of unforeseeable circumstances, or the result of the client's lifestyle.

Rethinking Root of the Problem

There are two types of factors I consider when it comes to what produced the inflammation, and they have to do whether they're in our control or not.

Factors Beyond Our Control

Genotype and genetic conditions, unexpected situations, or intensive medical procedures are inevitable in this peculiar journey we call life. Some of the most common include:

- **Structural or Physiological Differences.** Our bodies may be proportional but not necessarily symmetrical. Extremities or sit-bones could be off by a couple of millimeters or as much as one inch or more. The postural strain created when the differences are significant could go unnoticed for years until something seemingly benign crosses the threshold of tolerance. Correcting devices can mitigate this factor substantially. There are also structural inherited or genetic conditions such as Ehlers Danlos (EDS), Marfan syndrome, Chiari Malformation, Eagle's Syndrome, and Amyotrophic Lateral Sclerosis (ALS).
- **Blunt Trauma.** It's the most unequivocal trauma, and it results from mechanical forces exceeding tissue tolerances. Typical in accidents and sports injuries.
- **Infections.** The immune system response to intrusive elements elicits the response we know as infection, which generates high levels of inflammation. Infections could be acute, such as upper respiratory infections or food poisoning, or could be recurrent, such as Lyme. In a broader sense, I also include sensitivities to dietary and environmental factors such as gluten, mold, pollen, etc.
- **Surgeries.** Sometimes surgery is our only choice and while beneficial or lifesaving, it inevitably introduces scarring and/or foreign elements in the intervened areas. Consider also that surgeries are so common nowadays that we have forgotten how unnatural they are. The mechanics of routine surgeries would be lethal if it wasn't for modern medical technology. One should not expect a natural healing curve under those circumstances.
- **Intense Medical Interventions.** Certain life-saving procedures, such as chemotherapy, radiation, or prescription medications make efforts to be target-specific but it's virtually impossible not to have them affect our entire bodies. And it's not just the nature of the procedures, but also the intense biochemistry of anticipatory stress that patients usually experience.

Are the aforementioned beyond our control? I'd say that, given the choice, we would avoid them. What's difficult to avoid, though, is the inflammation those factors potentially generate, which could drive seemingly unrelated pains and dysfunctions.

Factors Within our Control

One of the shortcomings of claiming to address the root of the problem is that it exempts the client from their role. By making it appear as if the promoted method is the only solution, the responsibility is shifted to the therapist, thus making the disempowered client believe that only the purported method can get to the root cause and *fix* the problem permanently.

Reality says otherwise. Experience has shown me that the majority of factors producing significant inflammatory responses are self-inflicted. Consider some of the most common.

Segmental Overuse. Typical in manual traits such as carpentry, construction, electric work, knitting, etc. Also present in one-sided sports of high deceleration such as golf or racket sports; and common in seemingly benign activities performed for extended periods such as cycling, elliptical trainers, running, swimming, etc.

Postural Stress. Common when one spends significant time in the same position, whether seated or standing. Take surgeons, dental professionals, architects, drafters, and anyone involved in activities that require a degree of stillness for prolonged periods. Poor workstation ergonomics also force our bodies into less-than-ideal postures, which could compound to already existing mechanical stress from uncorrected structural differences.

Skewed Physical Fitness. There are those whose pursuit of strength, endurance, flexibility, and fitness makes them clash with our physiological and biomechanical limitations, which eventually express as chronic inflammation and strains.

Sedentarism. In my experience, sedentary individuals are virtually impossible to help long-term and their bodies seem to lack the ability to sustain therapeutic relief. The good news is that a little bit of activity goes a long way to deter the effects of sedentarism.

Respiratory Offenders. Industrial pollution, smoke, or vape matter drive inflammation. While one may think of the classic nasopharyngeal irritation symptoms, there are other seemingly unrelated symptoms such as neck and shoulder pain, costochondritis, lower back pain, brain fog, and/or migraines, that also result from respiratory offenders.

Poor Stress Management. Stress is a natural but brief response to help us protect our integrity or that of our loved ones, but becomes detrimental when chronically sustained.

Poor Sleep. This means more than not sleeping enough. There's consistency of sleep and wake-up times, understanding circadian rhythms, being aware of the events preceding bedtime, and more. It is during sleep that our bodies flush out inflammation from our brains. Constant disruptions will compromise our cognitive functions and promote central sensitization.

Poor Dietary and Hydration Habits. Cognitively, we're all aware of the importance of clean food and water, yet many of us neglect it for convenience, perceptual escape, or recreation. Popularly, the effects of this negligence are confined to aesthetics, energy fluctuations, and gastrointestinal issues. Yet the ensuing systemic inflammation is rarely considered despite having much greater implications, like damage to our gut microbiome, which has been implicated in the perpetuation of chronic pain via inflammation of the enteric division of the autonomic nervous system [44].

As I see it, the much-clamored root of the problem would be a tangible physiological factor that is independent of, and impervious to, the biochemistry of our perceptions or our environment, and it's fixable only by one specific approach. To my knowledge, the existence of such a factor remains but a claim.

Can You Treat [Insert Condition]?

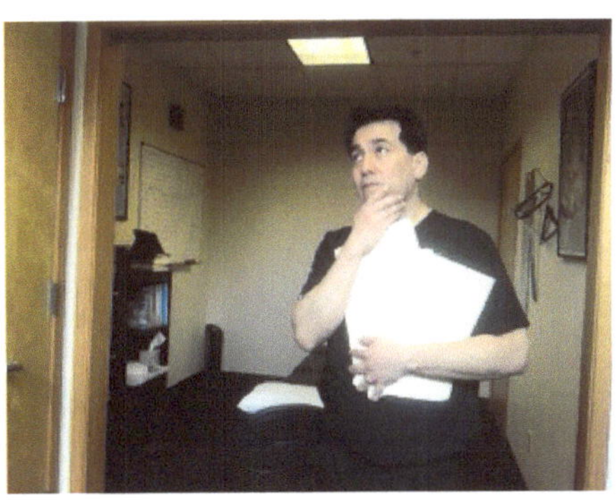

I'm in awe of the level of systemic orchestration and finesse that our daily activities require. Our bodies are amazing structures in which our multiple physiological systems interact not only holistically, but also independently for their specific functions, yet never separate from the whole.

That's what makes the following questions so difficult to answer in a soundbite format:

What conditions do you treat?

Or

Will Counterstrain be helpful for ... (insert condition?)

My answer is always, "I won't know until I start treatment."

At this point we understand that Counterstrain addresses trapped inflammation affecting multiple physiological systems simultaneously, thus, all dysfunctions could potentially have different sources. Further, the evolution of Counterstrain has morphed it into something far more powerful than a panacea for achy parts, and it is common for the advanced practitioner to see cases considered purely medical or even untreatable.

While I won't tell you that Counterstrain treats specific conditions, what I can tell you is that it has been immensely beneficial—if not the ultimate approach—in the successful treatment of many conditions. The following list is by no means definite and the conditions are listed in no particular order:

- Sciatica
- Lumbago
- SI joint pain
- Arthritis
- Migraines
- Tachycardia
- Dystonia
- Brain Fog
- Thoracic Outlet Syndrome
- Vertigo
- Postural Orthostatic Tachycardia Syndrome
- Radiculopathy
- Neuralgia
- Neuropathy
- Carpal Tunnel Syndrome
- Fibromyalgia
- Plantar Fasciitis
- Chronic edema
- Tinnitus
- Complex Regional Pain Syndrome
- Balance Issues
- Bell's Palsy
- Rotator Cuff Impingement
- Irritable Bowel Syndrome
- Chronic bloating
- Lymphedema
- Cervicalgia
- Seizures
- Peripheral arterial disease
- Chronic Fatigue Syndrome
- Visual disturbances
- Long COVID
- Post-Concussion Syndrome

I could not close this segment without mentioning that there are times when treating the chief complaint alleviates dysfunctions that were unknown to the therapist. Just because we address a specific problem, it doesn't mean the treatment won't have a positive effect on other issues, and the results, though remarkable, are unintentional.

Counterstrain Beyond Conditions

What brings clients to our practices are the conditions that nobody has been able to address. What keeps them returning is realizing that treating those conditions is only one dimension of Counterstrain therapy. Under the skilled care of a proficient practitioner, Counterstrain can be used as:

Preventive Medicine. Just as shedding cells, perspiration, and contact with environmental elements is a routine part of life, so is the production of inflammatory mediators. Just as we wouldn't wait until developing rashes or odors to shower and clean up, we shouldn't wait until the inflammatory stasis causes pain and dysfunction before draining it. And just as we would not expect one shower to keep us clean for the rest of our lives, we should not expect one session to keep the treated area permanently impervious to pain or dysfunction.

Prompt Relief When Taking Immediate Action. Counterstrain has been effective when applied immediately after evident trauma or acute idiopathic incidents. Provided there's nothing requiring dedicated medical care, Counterstrain can alleviate the severity of symptoms and optimize healing. When clients take an active part of their recovery it's not uncommon to reduce healing time from weeks to days.

Pre/post-surgery optimization. The nature of surgeries means that, through neural convergence, they will inevitably involve systems beyond their objective. As a modality that targets inflammatory stasis, Counterstrain can prepare the body by removing existing inflammation that could be exacerbated by the surgery. Counterstrain is also a welcome respite to the inflammation produced as the body heals post-surgery. Remember that as miraculous as surgeries are, they're still unnatural procedures that affect multiple layers of our physiology simultaneously, so high levels of inflammation should be expected.

Physiological-Perceptual Dysregulation. Thanks to advances in the understanding of our dynamic biochemistry, perceptual health is now recognized as a pillar of wellness instead of New Age quackery. Body and mind are inseparable, and perceptual issues manifest physically due to neural convergence.

The three key proinflammatory cytokines in Fascial Counterstrain, **Tumor Necrosis Factor Alpha** (**TNF α**), **Interleukin 1β** (**IL 1β**), and **Interleukin 6** (**IL 6**), are also present in *stress* [62]. Chronically stressed individuals are constantly activating the Hypothalamus-Pituitary-Adrenal (HPA) axis, which means they're constantly releasing norepinephrine, cortisol, and IL 6. This dysregulation shows up as elevated levels of epinephrine in the blood plasma and elevated IL 6 in the cerebrospinal fluid, [13] which should concern us since we now know what those mediators do when they stick around for too long.

I have found Counterstrain immensely valuable to help those experiencing Post-Traumatic Stress Disorder (PTSD) get the edge they need to maximize the benefits of their mental therapies as physiology and the perception must be addressed to find resolution and long-term relief. Dr. Holly Christy, ND, LAc, CACI, JSCCI, CSC I, published a breakthrough study on the significant benefits of FCS on PTSD symptoms in the *Military Medicine Journal*, [63] which I will cover in the nervous system segment.

Counterstrain has also been immensely useful during the powerful cytokine releases produced by grief. While the grieving process must be respected and allowed to run unobstructed, Counterstrain can make the physical manifestations of grief more bearable.

Finally, modern life seems plagued with chronic stress from work, the news, and routine surroundings, all of which create stealthy levels of inflammatory stasis that eventually compromise cellular health and manifest as mysterious pains or illnesses. As much as I'd love to say that the key to perceptual health is to mind our thoughts and reactions, I've come to learn that the factors creating our identity and idiosyncrasies are so embedded in us that they feel as normal as breathing, and as such, are hard to recognize or change.

Fortunately, there are now ample professional resources to help us figure out why we allow stress to dominate our perception, and what we can do to change it. The results of combining Fascial Counterstrain with mental health modalities have been promising and more research is currently being conducted.

Improved sleep. It's difficult to allow the body into the natural sleep cycles when trapped inflammation constantly sounds the alarm. Fortunately, the calming effects of Counterstrain can be felt immediately during therapy, and reports of deeper, more restful sleep post-therapy are common. But there is a catch. Counterstrain does not absolve us from the disruptions caused by chaotic perception, blue light, stimulants or depressants, or an irregular sleep schedule. As long as those factors are not addressed, sleep quality will continue being compromised.

Athletic Recovery and Sports Performance. Athletes who initially received Counterstrain to deal with injuries noticed how much their strength, flexibility, and stamina improved after their sessions so they started adding regular preventive visits. They were among the first to experience how regularly draining stagnant inflammation helped them not only perform better, but also prevent injuries and recover faster.

One of the freeing aspects of observing our physiology from the Counterstrain perspective is recognizing that just labeling a group of symptoms as a condition confines them to narrow parameters and obscures the larger picture because those symptoms are potential expressions of trapped inflammation. This has helped me look past the limitations set by accepted conditions and revamped how I assess my cases.

And no, Counterstrain is in no way substitute for professional medical care. When the pathology needs emergency medical care, surgery, medications, corrective aids or devices, or other professional medical treatments, no amount of Counterstrain will make a difference, and it may even be counterproductive. However, when the condition has been lingering and no evident driver or pathologies can be identified through medical studies, then the FCS assessment process can help us explore the factors that only Counterstrain can identify.

Now, before I tell you how I use the FCS assessment process, I want to make sure that you understand what it is that I'm looking for. For this, we need to appreciate how some of our physiological systems behave in the presence of inflammatory stasis. It's important to remember that while Counterstrain can help us get a more precise picture of physiological systems involved in a specific dysfunction and/or pain, it is in no way substitute for medical studies.

THE BODY SYSTEMS AND PAIN

I've been so immersed in the Counterstrain field that I usually forget how prevalent the musculoskeletal bias still is. Pain and dysfunction that did not respond to exercises, intensive manual therapy, or stretching continue their vicious cycle under other providers who continue with the same methods, as if repeating them would somehow render them effective.

This is what Tim Hodges meant when he talked about unlearning what we've been taught. It takes effort to master the dimension where hypertonic muscles, weak structures, postural deviations, and systemic dysfunctions are no longer the issues, but rather, the clues leading to the source inflammation.

This source inflammation is what Counterstrain therapists refer to when talking about their findings in different systems. You'll hear them mention vascular, neural, bone, or visceral structures many of which are unfamiliar to daily vernacular. And they won't be talking about pathology but rather, of that inflammatory stasis driving aberrant reflex arcs.

It's worth mentioning that it's extremely rare to work in only one physiological system for an entire session. The grand majority of conditions are a combination of multiple systems interacting with each other, and the source inflammation from each one has to be drained to find resolution to the problem. Take for instance, Irritable Bowel Syndrome (IBS) that showed up a couple of months after a gastric illness. Researchers now have evidence that this type of IBS can affect up to 36% of those who experienced a gastrointestinal infection [64]. Cases like this usually involve work in the viscera, but also in the visceral vasculature, not to mention the autonomic nervous system.

In case you're wondering whether we ever treat the musculoskeletal system, we do, but only when it harbors the source inflammation. Because of muscle guarding reflexes, the musculoskeletal system will always be involved as a reactive component. Under these circumstances, no amount of exercising, stretching, or pounding will make a difference.

Let us now get broadly acquainted with some of the physiological systems we indirectly treat in Counterstrain, and how they contribute to conditions we may have catalogued as orthopedic or idiopathic.

THE LYMPHATIC VENOUS SYSTEM AND PAIN

The module *Counterstrain for the Lymphatic/Venous System* has grown substantially since the first time I took it in April of 2013. What used to be one module is now two and their mastery is critical for successful therapy.

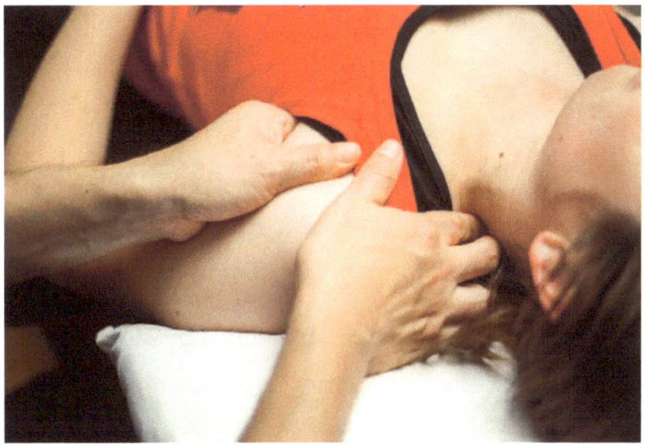

It's important to clarify that although it's still widely accepted that lymphatic flow depends on conscious muscular action, most of us do not wake up looking like frightened puffer fish after sleep inactivity. That is because the lymphatic system has engines of its own called *lymphangions*. They may sound familiar since they were mentioned when we reviewed how the lymphatic system increases its lymphangion activity in the presence of many inflammatory mediators [49]. These specialized structures get their motion from their layers of cardiac and smooth muscle which, combined with the smooth muscle layers of the larger lymphatic vessels, can move fluids independently [13] [65]. The importance of the lymphangions in fluid flow health is gathering attention as poor lymphangion health is being associated with congestive heart failure [66]. All lymphatic channels follow and connect with the veins, which start at the capillary beds and use shunts to move fluids to the liver and kidneys for filtration and eventually back to the heart.

However, movement and exercise are still important for overall fluid flow health. Keep in mind that the interstitium is a compressible and distensible pre-lymphatic structure whose pathways surround tissues involved in frequent movement such as the musculoskeletal system, lungs, and/or digestive tract [13] [32]. Theoretically, the dynamic nature of these tissues enhances the existing interstitial flow.

When it comes to dysfunctions, conventional therapy pays attention to the lymphatic/venous system only when dealing with systemic fluid irregularities, not in conditions such as radiculopathy, numbness, or brain fog. That is not so in Counterstrain. We take into account the presence of veins and lymphatic channels not only in the more accessible soft tissues, but also in our bones—including the spine—as well as medulla, dural layers, and cardiac fascia; and understand how disruptions driven by inflammatory stasis can manifest as musculoskeletal or systemic conditions. Fortunately, treating the larger vessels is more than enough to have a positive systemic effect.

Why Treat the Lymphatic Venous System?

When we say we're treating the lymphatic/venous system, we're not implying pathology. Rather, we are referring to IIS affecting the tunica adventitia of the veins—their most outer fascial layer. Unless the lymphangions or venous shunts have been damaged by infections or procedures, draining this inflammatory stasis can dissipate its related symptoms without the need of elevation, compression, or specific exercises.

A common instance is the resolution of bilateral (both-sides) pain after draining the inflammatory stasis from the spinal veins, which are usually affected by overuse, environmental pollutants, or certain medications. Counterstrain for the lymphatic/venous system has also proven effective in recovering from DOMS (Delay Onset Muscle Soreness) after intense exercise.

Many issues considered neural, such as weakness, tingling, and numbness in the extremities, can also involve the lymphatic/venous system in their spinal, visceral, or peripheral divisions. Common triggers tend to be dietary—as in certain food intolerances—as well as certain medications, and remnants of abdominal procedures. The lymphatic/venous system can also be involved in issues of frozen shoulders, thoracic outlet syndrome, and brain fog, which usually have the common factors of respiratory infections or whiplashes.

There are cases where the involvement of the lymphatic venous system seems obvious, such as bruising, discoloration, and edema, but the proficient Counterstrain Therapist knows that the lymphatic venous system is not the only one involved in these conditions and will only treat what is indicated by the assessment.

Mastery of the lymphatic/venous system is vital, as all of our techniques drain trapped inflammation. Even if not directly involved, the lymphatic/venous system must be constantly checked to ensure that the released inflammatory stasis is being channeled for elimination. Failure to do so may result in post-treatment malaise, flaring up systems that were close to the threshold of tolerance, and may even reduce treatment effectiveness. That's why all aspiring Counterstrain therapists are encouraged to master this module early in their careers and to pay attention to the updates.

THE VISCERAL SYSTEM AND PAIN

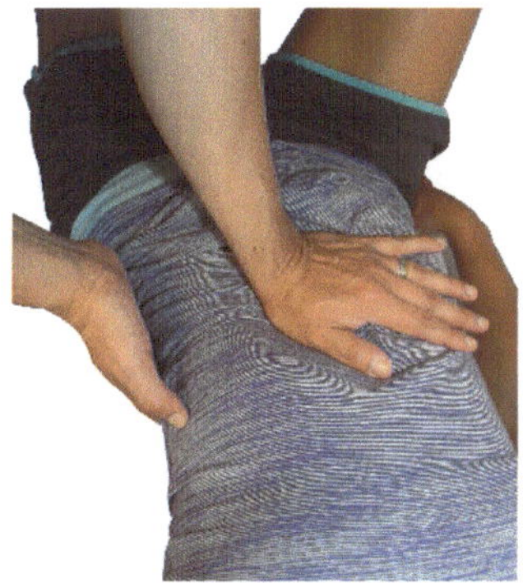

Visceral manipulation for medicinal purposes goes as far back as the beginnings of traditional Chinese medicine. However, it wasn't until the 1980s, when visceral manipulation received more attention thanks to the efforts of French osteopath Jean-Pierre Barral, who created a system of visceral treatment. Since then, many visceral therapeutic approaches have been developed.

Coming from a background of direct manual therapy, I first thought Counterstrain wouldn't have the reach of more established modalities, but my first meeting with Tim Hodges changed that. He did not speak of organ function per se, but of the physiology of the anchors that hold our organs in our cavities, and how they're affected by aberrant reflex arcs. While it all made sense theoretically, it wasn't until I witnessed the power of Counterstrain for the viscera in my practice that I was able to comprehend what Tim had tried to convey.

In all fairness, my previous direct visceral methods helped me in many complex cases, but many of the techniques were uncomfortable, more so if the client was overweight. That is not the case in Counterstrain, since the gentle but effective indirect work allows the client to let go of any apprehensions associated with direct visceral manipulation.

Will Counterstrain for the Viscera Impact Organ Function?

As stated earlier, the focus is not on the organs themselves but on their anchoring fascial sheaths. The majority of people whose issues are driven by visceral anchors come into our practices complaining of back or shoulder pain, not of organ dysfunction. While treating visceral anchors may not necessarily remove existing organ pathologies, organ-function improvements have been observed after, possibly because we're also influencing the enteric division of our autonomic nervous system.

Actual organ issues are multi-systemic. Consider the effects of IIS in the different divisions of the autonomic nervous system as they moderate organ function, vascular flow, and interaction. Treatment for the viscera may may be beneficial but not sufficient, since each division of the autonomic nervous system has its own treatment. Consider that organ issues can also be driven by vascular structures—which also have their own treatment—and you'll see why a proficient Counterstrain therapist will rarely equate organ pathology to visceral treatment without proper assessment.

Why Treat the Visceral Fascia?

The concept of visceral anchors influencing common musculoskeletal dysfunctions seems so bizarre that it confuses clients whose complaints were diagnosed as orthopedic. *You mean to tell me that my rotator cuff pain is actually lung fascia?* The skepticism vanishes after a couple of minutes of work, when the difference they're feeling settles their concerns.

Inflammatory stasis in anchors of the upper pleura (inner rib cage fascial lining) and pericardium (fascial heart sac) are common in clients diagnosed with tight scalenes. Many issues of uncorrectable slouching, shoulder pain, costochondritis, and upper back pain can be resolved by addressing upper digestive tract anchors, not to mention that the treatment can also help with swallowing, breathing, and reduction of GERD. Issues of thoracolumbar restriction, pain, and dysfunction attributed to paraspinal muscles can be successfully resolved by treating the lower pleural and diaphragmatic anchors. Stubborn issues of Sacroiliac (SI) joint pain, hamstring tightness, poor core mechanics, sciatica, lower extremity edema, and weak glutes can be helped by treating the upper and lower abdominal anchors.

Keep in mind that anything affecting the integrity of the thorax and the abdomen will also affect the visceral anchors. For instance, women who underwent C-sections or experienced perineal tears will present with idiopathic cases of sacrum pain, pelvic floor issues, or hamstring rigidity. Consider also excessive intraabdominal fat, or swelling of the abdominal cavities, which may require medical attention first before any Counterstrain therapy.

THE ARTERIAL SYSTEM AND PAIN

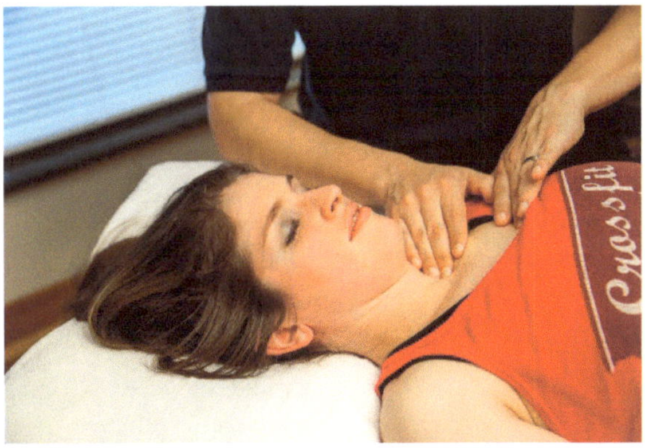

Just like the veins, the arteries have their own tunica adventitia but unlike the veins, the arteries have thick muscular walls to power blood transportation and its vital elements from the heart to all of our nooks and crannies.

A reminder: we're not dealing with pathology. A diagnosis of arterial treatment in Counterstrain has no direct involvement with elevated lipids, elevated glucose, or other typical blood markers. We are only referring to inflammatory stasis in the interstitium of the arterial tunica adventitia.

Just like in the veins, it's been observed that the major arterial vessels and their larger branches are involved in the protective response and draining their inflammatory stasis has a positive effect on the smaller vessels. Not only do we address the larger aortic branches supplying our neck, chest, abdomen, head, and extremities, but also the arteries supplying all spinal structures, all divisions of the nervous system, and even the cardiac fascia.

Why Treat the Arterial System?

The concept of arterial health can be traced as far back as the late 1800s, when Dr. Andrew Taylor Still, the founder of osteopathy, postulated: "*The rule of the artery is supreme... and must be absolute, universal, and unobstructed or disease will result.*" But it wasn't until the emergence of Fascial Counterstrain that this tenet could be put into practice.

The number of symptoms driven by inflammatory stasis in the arterial system can be expressed as DOMS, fibromyalgia, muscular tightness, or cramps. There are also issues where arterial involvement may not be as evident and can manifest as chronic migraines, tinnitus, vertigo, blurry vision, or TMJ. Many issues of joint pain—whether shoulders, knees, hips, elbows, etc.—and abdominal pain or rigidity, find resolution after arterial treatment.

The arterial system can also be involved in issues of poor perfusion, organ function deficiencies, and slow tissue restoration such as in tendonitis, fasciitis, osteoporosis, or post-surgical recovery. One of the most astounding cases I've ever reviewed came from Brian Tuckey himself, in which he was able to save his client's foot from amputation by applying arterial treatment [67].

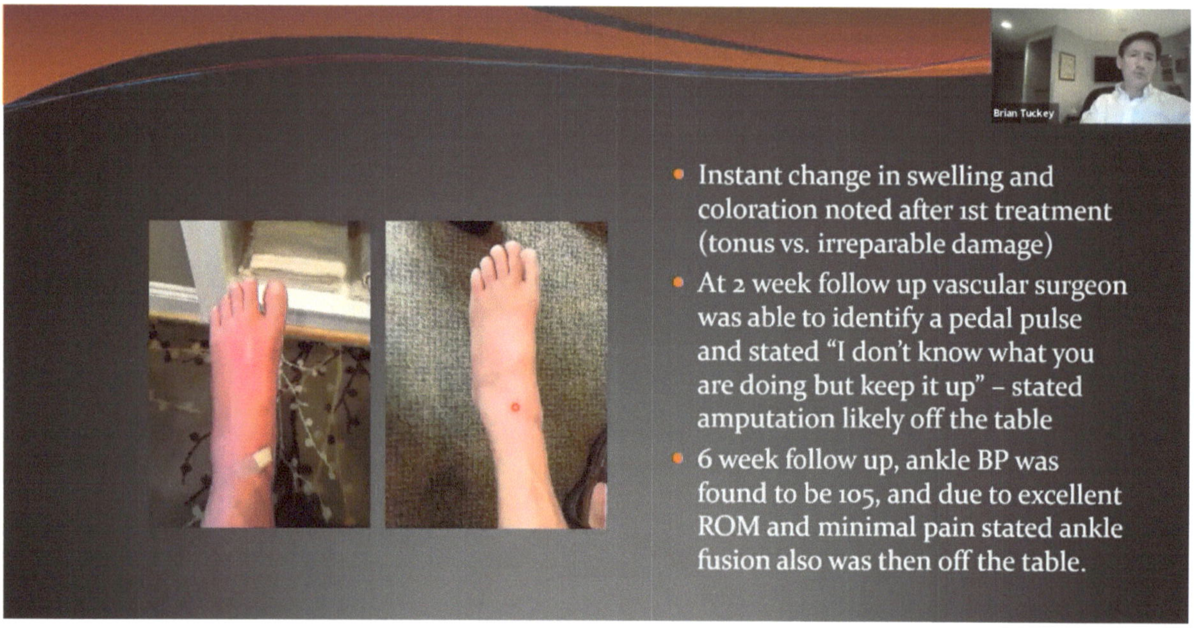

Brian Tuckey goes over the case of a patient whose foot was saved from amputation through FCS for the arterial system. The case is covered in the June 10, 2021 video "FCS 101: Headaches and Head Injuries" of the Jones Institute YouTube channel.

The effects of treating the arterial system are powerful. Clients report a substantial reduction of their discomfort, improved range of motion, reduced swelling, improved skin temperature and hue, improved organ function, improved tissue healing, improved recovery from tendonitis and fasciitis symptoms, and quite often, improved sports performance.

For the proficient Counterstrain therapist, the interaction of the lymphatic venous and arterial systems is a process we must honor to help our clients get the best outcome.

MUSCULOSKELETAL FASCIA AND PAIN

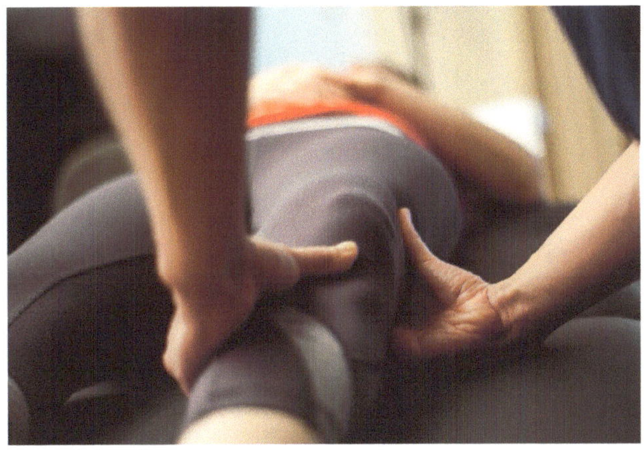

Because of the muscle guarding reflex, the musculoskeletal system will always be involved in all dysfunctions [45], which unfortunately obscures the roles of bones or cartilage in the issue unless they have been directly compromised. No therapist in their right mind would attribute intact shoulder cartilage as the driver of issues diagnosed as rotator cuff, or intact hip cartilage as producing sciatica. But intact doesn't necessarily mean functional or healthy. Said structures don't need to be damaged to harbor the inflammatory stasis that will inevitably affect the interacting musculoskeletal fascial layers and neighboring structures.

The Components of Musculoskeletal Fascia

It's impossible to discuss musculoskeletal fascia without considering how it flawlessly blends into the fascia of bones, cartilage, viscera, arteries, veins, organs, nerves, and brain structures. For this specific segment, we'll keep it at the four components we currently address in Counterstrain therapy.

Myofascia. Myofascia is skewedly the darling and culprit of all orthopedic issues because it is the more relatable of the fascial layers and it illustrates the concept of full body connection. One look at the works of Tom Myers helps us appreciate how restrictions in the calf or heel areas affect neck flexibility, or how one hip injury can affect opposite shoulder mechanics [68]. At the same time, myofascia can show us its immense influence as it interacts with the larger spinal ligaments. Thus, anything that affects myofascia has a disruptive potential on spinal ligaments, and anything affecting spinal ligaments could consequently affect myofascia.

Periosteum. The most external lining of the bones is rarely considered by the therapeutic and sports-performance communities, save the uncommon diagnosis of periostitis. But the lively and reactive periosteum is the seamless bridge to ligaments, cartilage, myofascia, viscera, vascular structures, neural structures, and brain structures. It should not surprise us, as bones are a key component of blood health, and primordial in organ response and survival responses [69].

Cartilage. It is common to find cases of sudden and unexplainable ACL (anterior cruciate ligament) issues to also have a history of meniscus (knee cartilage between upper and lower leg bones) injuries. Not really a mystery, since the meniscus and the cruciate ligaments (which includes the ACL) are one continuous structure. The same is true for issues of upper arm weakness that have a history of shoulder labrum (cartilage between the scapula and humerus) injury, since the labrum and long head of the biceps brachii are one continuous structure. The rabbit hole gets deeper when we start paying attention to mundane cartilage such as costal (rib) cartilage, sternal cartilage, temporomandibular joint (TMJ), and more.

Superficial Fascia. This membranous subcutaneous fascial layer is present in every region of our bodies, varying in thickness, elasticity, and fat content, depending on how much mechanical work the specific area has to exert [70]. This highly innervated layer is powered by the autonomic nervous system in both sympathetic and parasympathetic divisions, thus, playing a significant role in the perpetuation or alleviation of protective mechanisms. Dysfunctions in this structure can potentially compress superficial vascular structures, consequently impeding drainage, trapping inflammation, and triggering guarding responses.

Why Treat the Musculoskeletal Fascia?

While direct myofascial treatment has a well-deserved reputation, it's by no means infallible. I have observed it effective *when* myofascia is the driver, but *not* when the issues are driven by the broader spinal ligaments, cartilage, periosteum, or superficial fascia. This differentiation is crucial for successful treatment, as myofascial, cartilaginous, ligamentous, periosteal, and superficial fascial treatments are vastly different from each other in approach and sequencing.

Take, for instance, hip/pelvis stiffness, constipation, IBS, back pain, and neck pain, which manifest as common postural deviations. They all present similar symptoms and physical characteristics but may need different approaches depending on which of the musculoskeletal structures is affected and what other structures will show up as treatment progresses. It's not uncommon to start with myofascial treatment only to shift to spinal ligaments, and then back to myofascia, or other systems.

Minor dysfunctions in bone periosteum may not produce deformation but may be enough to alter the length-tension relationship of its attached structures. Treating such dysfunctions has proven helpful in relieving chronic hamstring and upper extremity tightness, upper and lower extremity weakness, reduced range of motion, minor limb-length differences, poor bone circulation, and calcic growths. Counterstrain for the periosteum also has calming effects in cases of acute or chronic anxiety, and it's an invaluable ally in the treatment of PTSD.

Spinal ligamentous treatment and cartilage treatment have shown benefits in issues of capsulitis, rigidity, chronic pain, and chronic inflammation. One of the most powerful treatments in this realm is to the ligamentum flavum in all spinal segments. The presence of IIS in the ligamentum flavum can cause hypertrophy that creates conditions typically blamed on spinal degeneration [71]. To this date, I don't know of any other therapeutic modality that targets the ligamentum flavum like FCS does.

A significant number of pain issues attributed to injured intervertebral discs can be helped by the application of Counterstrain, as draining the trapped inflammation from those structures helps them shut off the protective guarding mechanisms. Many studies have attributed intervertebral disc nerve endings triggered by inflammation as the drivers of pain rather than bulging or herniations. While the inflammation per se is a normal part of the disc-healing process [72] it is the inflammatory stasis that leads to chronic disc degeneration and pain perpetuation [13].

The combined work of musculoskeletal fascial layers is immensely helpful in cases of chronic systemic inflammation such as fibromyalgia, and also as an excellent preventive measure for sports injuries. For those who get regular maintenance treatment so they can perform at their best while minimizing injuries, the combination of Counterstrain for the musculoskeletal fascia and the vascular fascia is a winning combination.

THE NERVOUS SYSTEM AND PAIN

The nervous system seems to be the one area where all its ailments are already established. *Nerve pain*, *pinched nerve*, *nerve entrapment* and *phantom pain* are some of the most ubiquitous descriptions/diagnoses for a vast number of conditions.

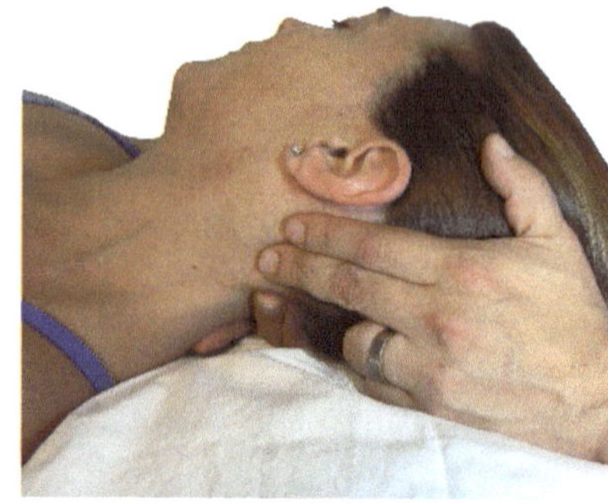

The issue is not whether the aforementioned are real. Those conditions do exist but are often attributed haphazardly, sometimes without medical studies, and even if studies are negative the diagnoses are still applied. After all, if it burns, numbs, radiates, or weakens, it *has* to be a nerve. I will acknowledge that every pain we feel is unequivocally a nerve signal, but it doesn't mean the dysfunction is in the actual nervous system, even if it feels like it.

The fascial layers of the nervous system that react to IIS are their epineurium and endoneurium [73]. While the nervous system reacts to the same sensory and mechanical stimuli as other fascial structures, it also deals directly with perceptions turning into physical responses.

Explaining the interactions of the different divisions of the nervous system is a worthwhile topic and there are fantastic textbooks on the subject. On my part, I'll focus on how popular views about the nervous system undermine the interactions of its divisions with the rest of our physiology. However helpful those views may be in illustrating the different divisions, they fall short in illustrating the integrated responses.

Central Nervous System

The Central Nervous System (CNS) is popularly viewed as the beginning and the end, the command center—if you will, of our lives. Broadly speaking, it consists of the brain and spinal cord, and I personally include the dural tube. While far more elaborate and capable than our most advanced computers yet developed, the CNS is more involved in environmental prediction and action, thus limited in a direct role during protective responses.

- **Brain.** When we think of the brain, we tend to focus on the components of its mass in a way that gives the impression that it's independent from its surroundings. We seem to disregard how the brain interacts with its meningeal layers, cranial ligaments, cervical and cranial bones, vascular, neural, and draining structures, auditory structures, optic structures, and more. Further, when we think of the brain, we generally think of gray matter or cortex, and rarely do we even consider the cerebellum or even the cranial nerves—any of which could generate a protective response without having to ask the brain for permission.
- **Spinal Cord.** The general view is that of a thick cord coming from the main command center, which then divides into the smaller peripheral cords to activate muscles and organs, or sense the environment. Seldom are pre/post ganglionic branches, gray/white rami communicants, spinal vascular structures, spinal ligaments, or glial cells considered, unless pathologies are involved.
- **Dural Tube.** A great deal of attention was brought to the dural tube and cerebrospinal fluid (CSF) mechanics, thanks to the contributions of craniosacral therapy, osteopathic medicine, and chiropractic medicine [74]. However, despite being a structure rich in nerve endings and multiple layers, the dural tube is still only seen as a contractile pouch whose main function is to house CSF. It seems that we have forgotten that the dural tube merges flawlessly with membranes—or meninges—that envelop the brain and its lobes, namely the falx cerebri and tentorium, and even upper cervical muscles. Understanding these interactions is crucial to address complex pains patterns.

Peripheral Nervous System

When popular view speaks of nerves, this is the division it usually refers to, mainly its **somatic division**, confining its function to voluntary movement. This popular view conceals the integrative nature of peripheral nerves as the bundles of neurons that consist of sensory and motor fibers for both voluntary and involuntary motion as well as *afferent* (toward the spine) and *efferent* (toward the periphery, organs, and vasculature) signals.

The sensory and motor nerves of the somatic division may work in harmony for voluntary movement when responding to an intention, but they are not necessarily responsible for the changes in tone, mechanical force production, or flexibility. Recall how our *protective reflex arcs* create immediate involuntary motion through musculoskeletal structures to protect us from injury. We also know that neurogenic inflammation affects motor neurons via *muscle guarding reflexes*, and how this manifests as musculoskeletal deficiencies that cannot be fixed through strengthening and stretching modalities.

And let's not forget that both *somato-sympathetic* and *visceral-sympathetic* reflexes also affect musculoskeletal function. It is, then, obvious that we cannot address the somatic division without considering the influence of the autonomic division.

Autonomic Division

The latest attention to the Autonomic Nervous System (ANS) is on its role in the realm of perceptions, and not so much on its influence in organ function or idiopathic pains, save some pathologies. Even in such cases, autonomic branches—most commonly vagal—are usually viewed in the same light as somatic branches, thus having their issues relegated to direct physical interference, a.k.a., *pinched nerve*.

Further, the interactions of the different divisions of the ANS have been polarized to the point where they're seen as exclusive from each other, or as one being more desirable than the rest, with treatments aiming at influencing their biochemistry to increment their dominance. But our ANS is far more interactive than this portrayal and a quick look at its divisions will help us understand why.

Sympathetic Division. The Sympathetic Nervous System (SNS) is generalized in its presentation as the *fight or flight* system, thus unfairly viewed as the bad guy in the play.

We cannot deny the effects of perceptual dysregulation. Take the effects of stress, which is the interpretation of a stimulus we perceive as a threat. The threat doesn't have to be tangible; we only need to sense it as such to accelerate our heart rate and breathing, tense our muscles, disrupt our digestion, and flood our bodies with powerful proinflammatory cytokines [62]. While it is true that the SNS is the main driver in those survival responses—which could be detrimental when chronically activated—it also has a crucial role in sexual health, digestive health, thermal regulation, among many others when balanced and regulated.

Parasympathetic Division. The Parasympathetic Nervous System (PNS) is generalized in its presentation as the *rest and digest* or *feed and breed* system. PNS dominance is regarded as sign of overall good health and many approaches are aimed in increasing PNS activation, mainly through the vagus nerve. But it's not that simple.

The typical understanding of the vagus nerve doesn't acknowledge its dorsal and ventral aspects, which serve different roles in the health spectrum. It's true that relaxation and social interaction are regulated by vagal structures, but so are terror, depression, and extreme physiological responses [75]. We are all aware of people whose hearts stopped as a reaction to a strong emotion. While the popular view blames the SNS, in reality it was the PNS that overregulated heart function in a process known as the *vagal paradox* [76] from overactivation of the vagal brake.

And there is the forgotten components of the PNS, which include cranial nerves III (oculomotor), VII (facial), and IX (glossopharyngeal) and S2-S4 sacral nerves. The vagus nerve is a key player in PNS function, but it works in conjunction with the aforementioned nerves as well as the SNS.

Enteric Division. The enteric nervous system (ENS) powers what we know as our gastrointestinal (GI) tract, and it's perhaps the least understood of all of our autonomic branches. Its complexity, complete autonomy from the CNS, and influence are so powerful that the ENS has come to be known as our second brain [77]. One could completely remove the GI tract from the abdominal cavity and it would remain in motion independently. The ENS communicates and influences the SNS and PNS divisions, and thus, also the CNS, not to mention that the ENS has its own communication pathways to the heart and brain. Let's not forget that inflammation to the ENS from altered gut microbiome has been linked to the perpetuation of chronic pain and dysfunction [44].

Fortunately for us, therapists, the entire nervous system is responsive to the principles and application of Counterstrain.

Why Treat the Nervous System?

What sort of symptoms does the presence of inflammatory stasis in the nervous system produce? That is highly dependent on which division of the nervous system is being affected.

For instance, inflammatory stasis in the abducens nerve—one of the twelve cranial nerves—can manifest as strabismus, headaches, or visual issues. Stasis in the hypoglossal nerve—another of the cranial nerves—may affect swallowing, speech, and may trigger upper cervical pain and headaches.

Inflammatory stasis in the thoracic division of the vagus nerve tends to show up as reflux, palpitations, postural distortions, and even depression. Chronic stress or severe emotional responses may flood the SNS division with inflammation [62], which then manifest as neck tightness/pain, digestive dysfunctions, palpitations, visual and hearing disturbances, shallow breathing, poor sleep, and symptoms usually attributed to organ insufficiency.

Inflammatory stasis in the peripheral nervous system usually manifest as muscular issues that respond poorly to exercise or mobility techniques. Many issues attributed to a weak rotator cuff group could be the result of IIS in the suprascapular, thoracodorsal, and long thoracic nerves, among others. The nervous system may also manifest dysfunctions that feel like tendonitis and even—gasp!—nerve pain and dysfunction. Many issues of neuritis, tingling, radiculopathies, and complex regional pain syndrome (CRPS) can be identified as IIS in the different divisions of the nervous system.

Clients with a history of concussions, skull fractures, facial and dental injuries, meningitis, whiplash injuries, cranial-based surgeries, severe allergies, and other conditions, usually exhibit central sensitization and require work in multiple CNS layers. This central sensitization usually manifests as chronic edema, digestive dysfunctions, impaired immune system, fibromyalgia, endocrine irregularities, neuropathies, chronic headaches, visual distortions, seizures, peripheral arterial disease, vertigo and balance issues, CRPS, tension headaches or migraines, facial sensitivity, photophobia—or sensitivity to light, tinnitus—or ringing of the ears, TMJ disorders, dizziness, neck pain, back pain, and others.

I could not conclude without mentioning how, in conjunction with mental health therapies, FCS has been immensely helpful in PTSD treatment. We did not intentionally set up to do so but it was revealed by many of our complex cases. Though they'd visit us for help with pain and dysfunction, they noticed their anxiety and depression dropping after their sessions, disclosing then their diagnosis. As Brian advanced treatments for the ANS and practitioners started reporting these observations, Dr. Holly Christy put the concept to the test. Her previously mentioned proof-of-concept study [63] highlights the power of FCS on reducing the severity of PTSD symptoms. Decreases in anxiety, depression, and improvements in quality of life in more than one factor were noticed in up to 80% of the involved clients, and improvements in at least one factor in 100% of the group that received treatment.

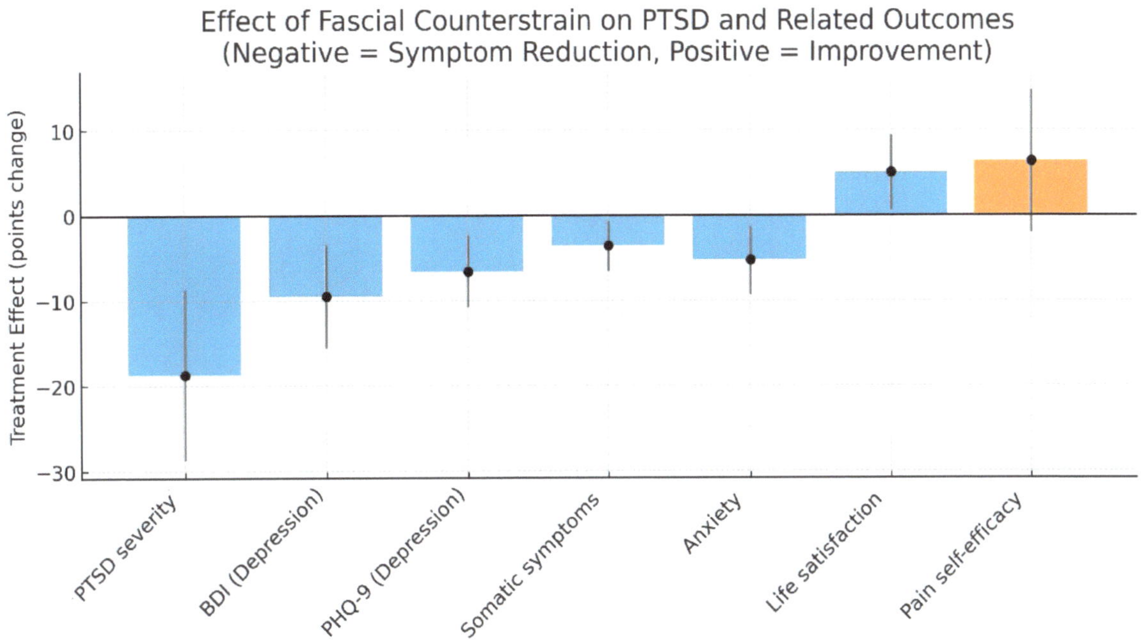

Results Compiled from Dr. Holly Christy's study published August 26, 2025, in the Military Medicine Journal.

It's encouraging to see that these changes were produced with no side effects, and the benefits were reported to last six months on average.

Counterstrain for the nervous system is one of the most demanding modules but also one of the most rewarding. Its mastery is a hallmark of all high-level practitioners, and mandatory for therapists wishing to pursue the newest, most advanced, and more complex FCS training.

WHAT ELSE IS BEING TREATED?

What I just presented is but a small sample of the systems we treat, most from the early days in my Counterstrain career. I also remember from those days how as our fascination with the fascial model grew, many therapists clamored for Brian Tuckey to finish his work so that a complete packageable system could be presented.

I'm so glad those days are long gone.

The more we learned and practiced, the more complex our cases grew—and the more stumbling blocks we found. This is what drove Brian's research, which ultimately led him to contemplate physiological systems that no branches of manual therapy had even considered.

For instance, when I originally took the Counterstrain modules for the lymphatic/venous and arterial systems, the emphasis was mostly on the peripheral and visceral vasculatures. As the client load grew in complexity, Brian analyzed the impact of dysfunctions in the vascular structures of the spine, identified their mapping in the cranial scan, and developed the corresponding techniques. At the same time, Brian noticed how his discoveries optimized and refined existing treatment. The refinements and updates were added to the curriculum, thus making it possible for all practitioners to be updated. While spinal vasculature has been extensively studied by the medical community, rarely is it considered as a factor of chronic pain in the manual therapy medicine field.

As Brian investigated more and received feedback from the instructors he trained, he ventured into physiological realms of great potential, some of which could be immediately used by students of every level. For instance, the work on contracted fibrosis, or **scar tissue**, resulting from the prolonged presence of inflammatory stasis, has become standard in all the new and updated classes.

But there are instances in which the latest discoveries can only be taught to the most advanced and dedicated practitioners. Consider how trauma, infection, interventions, or substances affecting meningeal layers or cardiac fascial layers—and their corresponding fibrosis from inflammation—can have a significant effect on the entire body or in areas in which impact from the aforementioned structures would never be considered. We're talking about treatment that addresses **central sensitization**, and it is, at this point, the most powerful series of modules in Counterstrain.

Since central sensitization can potentially impact entire physiological/organ systems, it can get reactive and unpredictable as its trapped inflammation is drained. The therapist must be ready to address any and all of those reactivities without hesitation. The confidence, knowledge, and experience required for successful central sensitization treatment demands in-depth development and training in our field.

Then there's the issue of being well ahead of the pack when it comes to recognizing issues in areas that conventional therapy ignores. Brian had recognized how IIS in the different expressions of adipose tissue perpetuated many orthopedic and central sensitization issues, and he developed the corresponding treatments. It's only now that the role of inflammation in adipose networks as a healing factor is starting to gather attention [78].

That's why I'm glad the days asking for a complete system are gone. Had the priority been put on commoditizing the system rather than exploring beyond what was already developed, the growth of Counterstrain would've stalled. Brian made it clear that as much as Counterstrain had grown, there was still a lot more growth left, and that something resembling a fully completed, packageable system was not even on the horizon. He also made it clear that his main concern was the accuracy of the system and that he wasn't going to compromise it for the sake of a few vocal individuals. It's been years since anyone has asked Brian when he is going to complete the system, and I seriously doubt anyone will ask again.

I believe this is an incredible time to be a Counterstrain Therapist. The system may not yet be complete, but it has a distinctive path and flow to guide therapists of all levels. To my knowledge, there are at least three new advanced modules in development, and the refinements and updates on the existing modules continue. Never have I been disappointed by any of the updates or additions to the Counterstrain curriculum, and I doubt I will ever be. The most enjoyable part of the new additions is integrating them to our existing repertoire, and this is possible thanks to our assessment methods, which we'll review next.

I'll say it again. What an incredible time to be a Counterstrain Therapist!

RETHINKING ASSESSMENTS

The way we find what we're looking for—meaning the source inflammation—is by identifying the distinctive physiological markers that IIS produces. Our FCS assessments are designed to take us precisely there, and quickly. This has dramatically changed how I assess in my practice. Whereas in the past I'd devote nearly thirty minutes to gather copious information and search for the root of the problem, I now devote between ten to fifteen minutes in the initial session, depending on case complexity. Assessments for follow-up sessions are even faster.

I conduct assessments with the understanding that they're a quick process that must be constantly repeated throughout the session as our bodies shift in response to treatment and reveal new information. This process took several years of studying and observing, which led me to the following conclusions:

- **Assessments are but Guidelines.** Because of life's innumerable confounding factors, assessments should be efficient in application and impartial in approach and interpretation. Lengthy or complex protocols could make therapists lose sight of the relationships between seemingly disconnected dysfunctions, or that the factors driving many mechanical deviations are beyond the therapist's control, or that they are harmless adaptations. For instance, an elevated shoulder with a rigid neck resulting from chronic stress cannot be helped long-term until the stress is managed. Take also those who have healed from fractures in their clavicular, scapular, costal, and iliac segments, and exhibit misalignments in the shoulders, thorax, and hip areas. While these adaptations may not be harmful, they could trigger pain when an alignment-obsessed therapist attempts to correct them.
- **Assessments Must Consider Individual Differences.** Differences in body, limb, skeletal proportions, and other variables, make it unreasonable to place everyone into tidy categories. And yet we still do, leading us to find dysfunctions where none exist. I frequently meet clients diagnosed with chronic tightness of the hamstrings/calves after they continually fail to break parallel in the standard squat. But there is no such tightness; rather, it's the clients' inherent mechanical proportions—long legs with long femurs, short shins, and a short torso—that give them a disadvantage in the standard squat. Adopting a wider stance with the toes pointing outward allows clients to squat to the desired depth and *fixes* the so-called tightness.

- **Assessments Should Minimize the Influence of Observation**. In general, the truer manifestations of movement, posture, and compensations take place when the client is unaware that they're being observed. This is virtually impossible when the client is being actively studied, which may lead them to conceal or exaggerate certain characteristics.
- **Assessment Results are Perishable.** One thing holds true regardless of the length of the assessment: *all the results and observations are temporary*. That's because our dynamic bodies start shifting as soon as the factors of therapy, relaxation, and expectation are introduced. This may not be immediately noticeable to the client, but it'll be evident to the therapist. Further, when therapy is properly sequenced, the body will continue unwinding and changing on its own for hours and even days post-session.

THE POWER OF THE COUNTERSTRAIN ASSESSMENT

I marvel at the evolution of Counterstrain and marvel even more at the advances and refinement of its assessment procedures. Nothing beats the time and sanity-saving qualities—for both the client and therapist—of the modern Counterstrain assessment methodology.

Witnessing the proficient therapist's fast but precise palpation that takes them forth and back from different segments of the body and then to the cranium until they zero in on a small but painful spot that the client didn't even know existed, is an experience in itself. No gadgets required.

But let's not confuse the process with the outcome, and that a proficient therapist makes it look easy doesn't mean that it was effortless to get there.

Consider the small sample of physiological systems we just overviewed. Full understanding of their components, integrations, and interactions with other systems not covered in this book is critical. But superb anatomical knowledge is only a component. Those aspiring for mastery must also develop the palpatory finesse that senses the presence of trapped inflammation, its changes during treatment, and also develop the interactive kinesthetic awareness that treatment positions unique to Counterstrain demand.

Therapists who came to Counterstrain with an in-depth anatomical background but ordinary palpatory skills struggled when they could not perceive the subtleties that make assessments accurate and allow us to monitor treatment. Others who came with a great set of hands but basic anatomy also struggled when the anatomical knowledge and motion-testing skills crucial in FCS were beyond what they had in their former professional curricula. That's what makes the FCS assessment process virtually impossible to copy. The behind-the-scenes view is detailed in Brian Tuckey's latest article, in which he goes over the governing principles in our methodology [26].

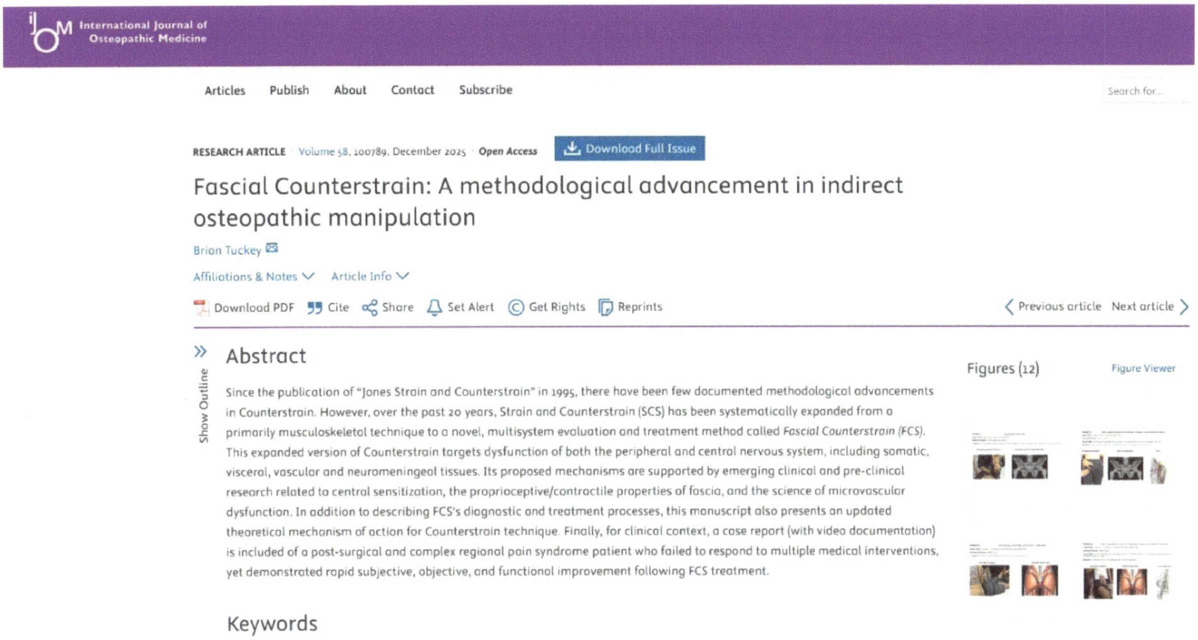

International Journal of Osteopathic Medicine

Articles Publish About Contact Subscribe

Search for...

RESEARCH ARTICLE · Volume 58, 100789, December 2025 · Open Access · Download Full Issue

Fascial Counterstrain: A methodological advancement in indirect osteopathic manipulation

Brian Tuckey

Affiliations & Notes · Article Info

Download PDF · Cite · Share · Set Alert · Get Rights · Reprints · Previous article · Next article

Abstract

Since the publication of "Jones Strain and Counterstrain" in 1995, there have been few documented methodological advancements in Counterstrain. However, over the past 20 years, Strain and Counterstrain (SCS) has been systematically expanded from a primarily musculoskeletal technique to a novel, multisystem evaluation and treatment method called *Fascial Counterstrain* (FCS). This expanded version of Counterstrain targets dysfunction of both the peripheral and central nervous system, including somatic, visceral, vascular and neuromeningeal tissues. Its proposed mechanisms are supported by emerging clinical and pre-clinical research related to central sensitization, the proprioceptive/contractile properties of fascia, and the science of microvascular dysfunction. In addition to describing FCS's diagnostic and treatment processes, this manuscript also presents an updated theoretical mechanism of action for Counterstrain technique. Finally, for clinical context, a case report (with video documentation) is included of a post-surgical and complex regional pain syndrome patient who failed to respond to multiple medical interventions, yet demonstrated rapid subjective, objective, and functional improvement following FCS treatment.

Figures (12) · Figure Viewer

Keywords

What I'll present to you is the procedures in my practice. They're based on the latest updates to the system but, like other therapists, I adapt them to the demands of my practice. This means that there might be slight variances in how other practitioners take medical history, motion test, and perform the cranial scan, but rest assured we all follow the same principles.

Medical History

The most difficult part of gathering medical history is removing the noise that the client has been inundated with. The information I prioritize and care about is where they feel their pain, when it started, what sensations they feel (whether it makes sense to them or not), and what makes the pain better or worse. I also care about their lifestyle choices, medical interventions, history of systemic conditions, and any long-term conditions they're getting treatment for.

The whole process takes ten to fifteen minutes on average. I need only to absorb the most salient points for the initial session and the rest of the pieces fall into place as I review the documents in between sessions. I might also make notes of candid postural and gait markers and document obvious restrictions before proceeding with motion testing.

Motion Testing

"I've got new ears, y'all!"

FRIEND OF MINE

This memorable line was blurted by a friend upon getting hearing aids and rediscovering the joy of listening to the sounds of nature he didn't know he'd been missing. It's notable because it signals an epiphany in a sensory experience.

There are moments where life reveals how oblivious we were to what we were lacking because we got used to lacking it. It's something I constantly witness when clients have had their restrictions for so long that they've been normalized. Imagine their astonishment not only when the restriction is brought to their awareness, but also of the post-treatment difference. Feeling the natural looseness and increased range of motion of their spine and limbs is like a gift and a revelation. They can move better, talk better, and hold an upright posture without straining.

The purpose of motion testing in Counterstrain is to narrow down the location where the inflammatory stasis has the most effect—the source inflammation. What we are looking for is summarized with the acronym **TART** [26].

- Texture abnormalities
- Asymmetry
- Restricted range of motion
- Tenderness

Depending on the condition and location of dysfunctions, I'll have the client sit or lie down on my treatment table and I'll start testing different segments to check for their restrictions and relationships. In general, the more restricted areas harbor the most TART, thus, the most significant dysfunctions. Motion testing is combined with *touch inhibition testing* to determine which of the involved structures harbors the source inflammation, and which are only expressions of retrograde inflammation. Touch inhibition is one of the most reliable tools in our assessment arsenal and, like other aspects of FCS, it feels magical but can be scientifically explained [26].

The efficacy of touch inhibition testing is theorized to be governed by another type of sensory neurons known as *Wide Dynamic Range Neurons* (WDR), which are found in the sensory area (dorsal horn) of the spinal cord [79]. In addition to converging with nociceptors, they also converge with neurons that detect mechanical, thermal, and chemical stimuli. This allows them to generate specific responses to a variety of inputs, which includes touch, which we in turn use to determine the location of the source inflammation.

Once the source inflammation is drained, the protective reflexes creating restrictions shut off and the TART dissipates. The affected segment is then retested. While it's rare for a single release to restore full motion—though it happens—the next most likely scenario is that while the joint may have improved its motion, the direction of its restriction will have changed. The therapist will then reassess to identify the next structure in the sequence.

Motion testing is widely used by orthopedists, osteopaths, chiropractors, physical therapists and other therapeutic bodywork professionals. It is also an excellent guide for acute cases or for circumstances when a complete evaluation is not possible, but it may be too broad for complex cases. There will be times when the area in pain has no restrictions or when a restricted area harbors no pain. There'll also be times when there will be so many possibilities in the affected segments that the therapist won't know what to prioritize.

This is where the next component of the FCS assessment process shows its power. As I mentioned earlier, seeing it in action and experiencing it under the guidance of Brian Tuckey was a life-changing event. It is the Cranial Scan.

The Cranial Scan

The cranium, or skull, is the subject of multiple studies but also of controversies and heated debate among therapeutic schools. I'm not here to favor or discredit any but to present the information as it pertains to Counterstrain.

We do treat the cranium but also use it as a critical component of our assessment arsenal. Since the cranial scan shows only the areas of source inflammation, not the areas of retrograde inflammation [26], it helps us refine our findings by identifying what system is affecting the rest of the systems and the priority and sequencing of treatment. This accuracy is a must for complex cases.

Let's examine a typical sacroiliac (SI) joint pain case where the SI joint is painful and inflamed but mobile. That means the pain is driven by dysfunctions elsewhere. My earlier observations and the client's medical history make me suspect the lumbar spine. Motion testing confirms TART at the L4 and L5 segments. Though the client does not complain of lumbar pain, the area is rigid and loaded with tender points that make the client wince. Fine-tuning my motion testing allows me to narrow down my findings to three possible systems.

I then go to the cranial scan to verify my findings, which shows only two of the systems. I discard the non-scanning system, as there's a high likelihood that its tender points are driven by another system. Next, I use touch inhibition to determine which of those two systems is driving the protective mechanisms.

Once I determine the driver, I'll fine-tune the cranial scan to verify the location. Since only the dysfunction at L4 shows up on one side, I go to that location to verify via motion testing, tender point palpation, and touch inhibition. I will then use the corresponding FCS techniques to drain the source inflammation restricting L4. When I'm finished, L4 moves freely and the tender point is gone, but I'm not done. Motion testing now indicates that L5 is still stuck but on the opposite side. The cranial scan and touch inhibition confirm my observations and show me that the same system is involved but in a different segment.

Once I free L5, the entire lumbar spine regains its mobility and no other systems or tender points remain but I'm still not done. I redirect my attention to the SI joint, which is now rigid. There is only one major tender point and the cranial and touch inhibition confirm it. One minute later, the dysfunction, pain, and inflammation are gone, and the SI joint moves freely.

The process I just described usually takes me around five minutes. That doesn't mean that all the issues are resolved but rather that the treated segments no longer harbor trapped inflammation. Depending on the age of the client, the length of time they've been dealing with the issues, medical history, and lifestyle choices, the remaining work could be only a few more releases or a few more sessions.

The uncanny but precise nature of the cranial scan baffles those who experience it. As much as the skeptics paint it as a show of metaphysics, the principles governing the cranial scan are science-based. And no, they're not the linear, one-answer-fits-all type of principles because the roots are multiple. Just as he did to develop Fascial Counterstrain, Brian Tuckey explored the common ground in seemingly unrelated fields including neurology, physiology, embryology, tensegrity, and osteopathy, in addition to his diverse education and experience in manual therapy, to arrive at the cranial scan principles. Though the exact mechanisms of the cranial scan have not been fully determined, they appear to be an expression of the IIS loop affecting the periosteal layer of the cranial dura [26].

One of my fellow teaching assistants traces the beginnings of the cranial scan to the time Brian was developing *Fascial Counterstrain for the Viscera* module. Brian was exploring the area where the cranial nerve that influences visceral health exits the cranial vault, and noticed that manipulating the visceral anchors produced palpable changes in texture and mobility in this region. If you recall my first Fascial Counterstrain class, then you know that I'm referring to the mastoid process, where the vagus nerve exits its uppermost posterior part via the jugular foramen. Brian discovered that all the corresponding visceral tender points were mapped in the area, and that the changes produced by the application of the corresponding Counterstrain techniques were a reliable indicator of treatment progress.

The rest is history, as Brian applied the same principles to other physiological systems and discovered that they were also mapped in different regions of our craniums. Subtle changes in the texture and feel in micro-locations within those regions corresponded to the presence of protective reflex arcs driven by inflammation, thus, draining the source inflammation restores healthy cranial texture and feel. This is a phenomenon that's been reliably observed by hundreds of practitioners in thousands of cases.

Every single one of the physiological systems we previously overviewed—and the ones we didn't cover—has a region in the cranium where their dysfunctions can be determined.

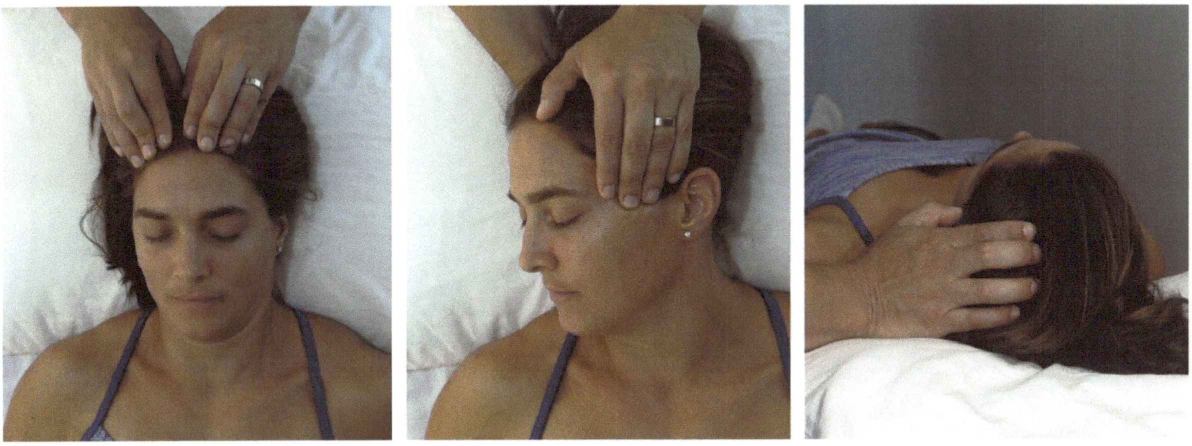

Example of cranial regions where different physiological systems are represented. Changes in texture and feel in these regions help determine the location of the source inflammation.

Further, each system has also its own micro scan where dysfunctions in their subdivisions are mapped. Remember the nervous system? For starters, the somatic nerves scan in their own micro regions. Where you scan upper body nerves is different from where you scan lower body nerves. Where you scan nerves in the front of the body is different from where you scan nerves in the back of the body. How you scan nerves in the sympathetic division is different from how you scan nerves in the parasympathetic division. Even subdivisions of the autonomic nervous system—such as white rami, gray rami, preganglionic, postganglionic—have their own scan in their own micro regions. Add the same level of detail to veins, arteries, viscera, myofascia, adipose tissue, collagenous connections, periosteum, etc., and you can see why the cranial scan is a crucial part of our assessment process.

There are, however, instances in which the client's condition may throw off assessment observations, and we'll discuss the topic as we cover assessment sequence.

Assessment Sequence

The aspect of Counterstrain I enjoy most is the absence of cookie-cutter protocols, which gives the therapist immense freedom to adapt the sequence of assessment to the specific needs of the client. In general, the TART identification sequence most people experience is motion testing, restriction and tender point identification, followed by cranial scan verification, source inflammation drainage, and reassessment.

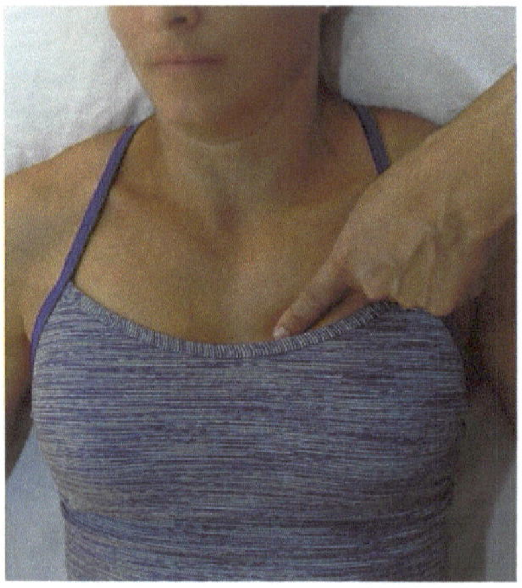

Motion testing and tender point palpation zero in on a dysfunction.

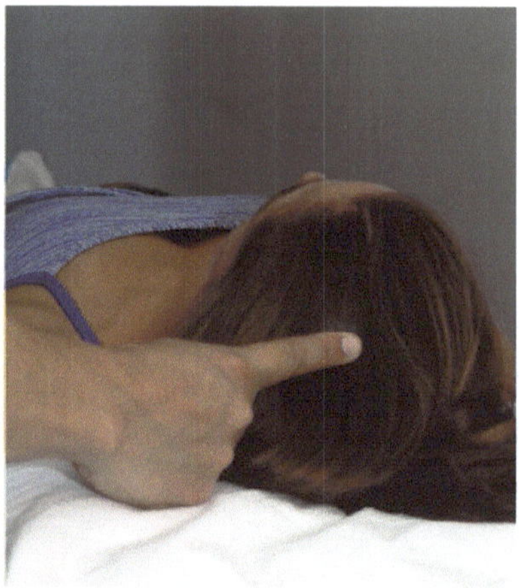

The location and system involved are verified via the cranial scan.

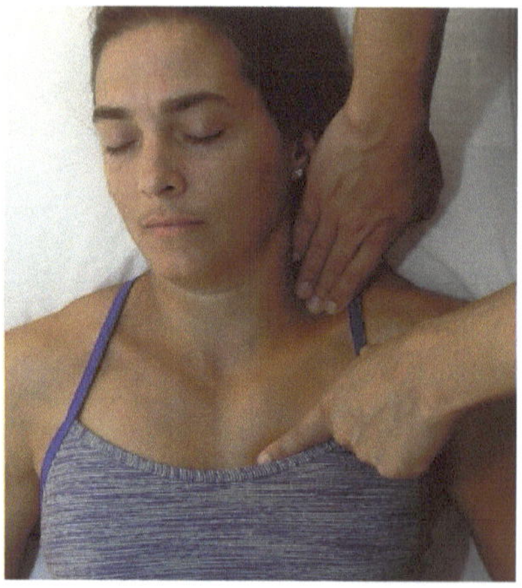

The therapist drains the structure and rechecks motion and scan to verify.

While this sequence is effective for general cases, it can be frustratingly unproductive when the client is experiencing **central sensitization**. That means inflammatory stasis in the central nervous system, which then affects multiple systems simultaneously. These clients exhibit myriad tender points that don't respond to treatment, or have no tender points but are in pain, or have tender points that won't show up in the scan. It's not unusual for such clients to exhibit cranial rigidity and distention.

Until the inflammation driving central sensitization is drained, motion testing and conventional cranial scan results will be unreliable. Fortunately, most Counterstrain therapists are now trained to identify this phenomenon via specific cranial scan and touch inhibition tests. Contingent on the therapist's level of training and experience, they may be able to address this issue themselves, or they may need to refer the client to more advanced practitioners.

Additional Assessments

Depending on the documentation required, specific procedures dictated by their practice, or comparative markers, Counterstrain therapists may add components to their assessment process. The addition or absence of such will have zero effects on the application and results of Counterstrain but may provide tangible comparative scenarios.

Range of motion testing for instance, can help therapists and clients appreciate the changes taking place as therapy progresses. Whether done via goniometer or visually, both therapist and client can have immediate feedback for documentation and comparative purposes. I alternate between goniometer and visual testing depending on the case. It's not necessarily numbers what I'm after, but rather, pain-free and unrestricted motion that the client can notice immediately.

Another widely used assessment is segmental strength testing. The ability of the affected segment to resist or produce mechanical force in specific positions is tested before and after treatment, or in the case of the more proficient therapists, during every significant release. While this process rarely employs linear measuring devices, the client's ability to exert more control of the affected segment after treatment can be unequivocally felt by both the client and the therapist.

It's worth mentioning that increased strength in an affected segment is usually accompanied by increments in range of motion. On the same line, any post-treatment improvements in range of motion are usually accompanied by increased control and strength in the affected segment.

Why the Assessment Is Crucial

There's a fact that those who forgo the assessment in favor of the techniques fail to understand: *all of the Counterstrain techniques can be rendered useless—and even counterproductive—when not sequenced properly*. The precise but dynamic hierarchy that dictates treatment sequence can only be determined during assessment. Anything less is a negligent guessing game.

Just because a proficient therapist successfully released thoracic rigidity by treating the post-ganglionic branches of the sympathetic nervous system doesn't mean that every case of thoracic rigidity will be treated as such. The proficient therapist targeted the aforementioned only because their assessment indicated it as the priority in the sequencing hierarchy. At the same time, the proficient therapist knows that maneuvering the sympathetic branches without following the sequencing can result in an imbalance that may lead to panic attacks, tachycardia, shortness of breath, digestive issues, and more.

It's no accident that the Jones Institute and the Counterstrain Academy place a high emphasis on assessment in their modules, and the workshops presented at the Counterstrain Conventions emphasize the assessment components. It used to be said—back when I started my Counterstrain career—that there's no such thing as bad Counterstrain, and that even bad Counterstrain is better than no Counterstrain. The latest advances show us that's no longer the case, since we're dealing with the dynamic interactions of all our physiological systems as they respond to trapped inflammation.

Every proficient Counterstrain therapist honors the importance of the assessment procedures and spends considerable time honing those skills. They know that's the key to helping their clients in the most efficient and safest way possible.

COUNTERSTRAIN AND YOU

Let me reiterate the following: *Though Fascial Counterstrain may share some commonalities with other approaches, it ultimately is an indirect healing modality that needs to be experienced to be fully understood.* Only then can we understand how its proprietary methods narrow the broad down to the specific in realms not considered in manual therapy.

This is determined by identifying the affected physiological system via the cranial scan, and its inflamed structural proxy or diagnostic tender point. The absence of any of those components is only manual therapy, but not Counterstrain.

Understanding Counterstrain

There are factors all proficient Counterstrain practitioners share. We're all in love with our field, we're hungry for knowledge and mastery, and while our quirks determine the flavor of our practices, we all honor and follow the same treatment principles.

The following are not rules but perspectives to help you make the most out of your Counterstrain experience.

Let Go and Let it Be

It is normal to look for a frame of reference when facing a new concept. Sometimes we find a frame that is so similar that it facilitates absorption of the new concept. But sometimes the new concept is so different that all frames of reference collapse, and in an effort to understand it, we force it into established models.

That is the case with Counterstrain, a modality that is its own entity in rationale and application. For those immersed, the principles, flow, and character of Counterstrain are so second-nature that we often forget how bizarre it seems to those outside our niche.

It's not uncommon for newcomers to compare it to craniosacral therapy, phrenology, reflexology, PNF, or even energy medicine. Others compare it to myofascial release or Rolfing the moment they hear "fascial involvement." It is at this point that I encourage these newcomers to *let go and let it be,* as their time and energy will be better served by wiping their slate clean, or better yet, getting a brand-new slate. Avoid comparisons or conclusions until you get feedback from your therapist because ...

What Seems to Be Isn't

Attempting to fit the novel into the familiar without first understanding what we're trying to fit in inevitably results in misconceptions. These misconceptions can range from exasperating distractions to detrimental applications when left unchecked.

A typical example took place when a client experienced a severe setback shortly after our first session. In inquiring about the circumstances leading to his flare up, he mentioned that the stretches I did on him during his initial treatment had made him feel so good that he tried to reproduce them on his own. Needless to say, I was puzzled since stretching is never part of treatment, and those who know me know of my loathing for the established approach to stretching. However, after a second, I knew what he meant.

It was then that I clarified that I never stretch anyone, and that every maneuver and position during treatment is aimed at indirectly creating slack in a specific structure, which will inevitably lengthen other structures. The main difference is that since I was going in the direction of ease, his body collaborated and the applied technique felt good.

That's why I always emphasize the rationale of trapped inflammation. This distinction is crucial in understanding Counterstrain in a world where direct manipulation of palpable/relatable structures is considered essential for treatment because ...

The Target may Be Intangible but its Effects are Not

Aberrant protective reflex arcs is a hard topic to illustrate without resorting to heavy scientific language or physiological structures whose names are not part of everyday vernacular.

But that was what we had to do until the role of IIS as the driver of the aberrant protective reflex arcs was revealed. Though the topic of inflammation is widespread, its physiological interactions are not given equal attention. Not surprisingly, clients wonder if it's truly inflammation: *How come anti-inflammatories have no effect?* (It's in the microvasculature, not in the bloodstream.) *Why can't it be controlled by anti-inflammatory diets?* (It's in the microvasculature, not in the bloodstream.) *How come it cannot be seen in imaging studies?* (Conventional imaging does not target the interstitium.) *And where does all that inflammation go after treatment?* (You pee it away.)

Just because the notion of aberrant protective reflex arcs driven by IIS may feel spectral, its effects are not. Muscular knots, rigidity, stiffness, weakness, pain, headaches, IBS, brain fog, etc., are all unmistakable and undeniable experiences that result from inflammation trapped in the interstitial spaces of a specific structure. It's not until that structure is identified and drained that one shuts off the dysfunction and relieves the symptoms.

This is important to keep in mind because when it comes to Counterstrain …

The Body is Always in Charge

Most Counterstrain novices experience such remarkable changes that they request longer or more frequent sessions. But that's not necessarily how Counterstrain operates, and session length and frequency are dictated by the clients' condition, their overall health, and the therapist's experience.

Since our goal is to drain trapped inflammation, there will be chronic complex cases with years of accumulation. The gentleness of Counterstrain may give the impression that it's easy on the body, but the drainage process has the potential to become taxing. Experience has taught me that the body starts signaling when it's approaching its limits and needs to be left alone so that its greater intelligence can take over. Any farther past that threshold, there's a significant chance that the client may experience severe post-treatment malaise. I'll go over it in more detail when we discuss post-treatment effects.

So, how long does it take for the body to reach that threshold? It all depends and I can only speak from my experience.

Most typical orthopedic cases—think minor strains, sprains, minor falls or accidents, minor infections, and most pre/post-surgical care—can be taken care of in one hour. Cases involving more severe injuries, systemic dysfunctions, major infections, autoimmune conditions, perceptual dysregulation, or central nervous system injury—such as whiplashes or concussions—usually require two hours or longer. Then there are the younger, fitter, and healthier populations with no major medical history who may need as little as a half-hour.

Currently, my services are one hour and longer. I used to offer shorter sessions but that was when I only had a handful of physiological systems under my belt. I could cover a lot of ground quickly, which meant the body would also reach its threshold quickly. Fast-forward to the present, and the astonishing evolution of Counterstrain has revamped my approach.

The impacts of trapped inflammation via neural convergence means that when we treat we must allow the affected structure to fully drain. This process may be swift (usually fifteen to forty-five seconds) in straightforward cases but the presence of fibrosis, neuroinflammation, or a combination thereof means that the pool may be more substantial and will take longer to drain, usually three to four minutes. This is the reason I discontinued shorter sessions. Clients started to flare up from the incomplete work as I ran out of time. But shorter sessions can still be highly beneficial for the right populations, and under those circumstances I refer to other practitioners.

Then there's the question of frequency. *How soon should one get a follow-up session?* Again, that is dependent on the specifics of the client. The body must be allowed to rebalance after treatment so that it can incorporate the changes and reveal any other possible dysfunctional layers. In simpler cases this usually takes place in seven to ten days. For more complex cases, or in severe acute pains and dysfunctions, this can be between one to five days. Adding more treatment without allowing the systems to reconfigure could prove overwhelming.

Once the most significant dysfunctions are addressed, and barring unpredictable circumstances (as in new injuries or illnesses), most clients return for a tune-up every four to six weeks. The caveat in those returning for maintenance is ensuring that they embrace their role and do not become dependent on Counterstrain as their sole means of relief because …

There are Perpetuating Factors

Perpetuating factors can be self-inflicted, or a byproduct of incomplete therapy, or congenital factors that are not evident until assessment.

Some of the most common self-inflicted perpetuating factors are poor dietary choices [80], alcohol consumption, smoking, vaping [81], poor sleep [82], sedentarism [83], poor posture [84], and/or chronic stress [62]. The physiological dysregulations they cause are detrimental to the body and to the healing process. It can be argued that the effects of inflammatory stasis do not discriminate between healthy and unhealthy individuals, but practical experience has shown me that those who neglect their health experience more pain, more dysfunction, and take much longer to recover than their healthier counterparts.

Then there's what happens when therapy is incomplete. Many older clients with decades old dysfunctions get discouraged when their pain is not fully resolved immediately and stop treatment prematurely. They may understand that the length of their dysfunctions has created compensatory mechanisms, but rarely do they understand that the body won't grant us access to the main dysfunction until we clear the compensatory layers. Then there are those who feel so good after a session that they stop altogether, even when they're recommended to follow up.

Both instances leave untreated layers that could create more neurogenic inflammation, which could potentially rekindle the original complaint or manifest as the reemergence of old conditions. Thus, it's not unusual for a client who discontinued their back-pain treatment to re-experience the hip pain they had forgotten about, or for the neck to revive whiplash pain once elbow and shoulder pains start to feel better.

There are also some conditions within the client that although not evident, can be identified by a therapist. Issues such as leg length discrepancies, small hemipelvis, or reactions to allergens need corrective devices or medical intervention. When left unchecked, they may become perpetuating factors. This is important to understand because …

Healing is a Partnership

Let's keep one thing straight. I *cannot* fix anyone, nor can I heal them.

My role in life is that of a healer, and it doesn't mean I provide with the healing but rather, I prepare the environment and remove the obstructions so that the body can do its own healing. Thus, the two of us work together for this purpose, and we do so in partnerships. There are two partnerships to keep in mind:

- **Between You and Your Therapist.** Though the visit to your Counterstrain therapist may only comprise a fraction of your weekly schedule, rest assured that all proficient therapists train and study exclusively to be able to go exactly where your body needs it. We're talking thousands of hours of training and practice—not to mention significant investments of funds and resources—that manifest as confident skills. On the one hand, your therapist commits to keep learning, training, and improving. On the other hand, you commit to following your therapist's recommendations, and not interfere with their work.
- **Between You and your Body.** This is, without a doubt, the most difficult of the partnerships. Know this: *Healing is virtually impossible without your cooperation.* That means to not only be cognizant of your therapist's recommendations, but also of lifestyle choices that derail the healing process—the perpetuating factors in your control we previously mentioned. When neglected, they will ultimately nullify the work done.

Keep the above in mind if your healing is not going as you expect it. I can guarantee you there's an area where a bit of improvement—whether it's something you should've done or should *not* have done—can go a long way in optimizing your healing.

HOW MANY SESSIONS WILL IT TAKE?

It seems that we have forgotten—or may not even be aware—that the number of sessions recommended for manual therapy is dictated by insurance guidelines rather than by physiology or the client's unique circumstances.

Fortunately, our bodies are resilient and even a few visits can be sufficient for straightforward cases, such as post-surgical recovery or most sports injuries. When it comes to idiopathic, chronic, or recurrent pain and dysfunction, however, determining the amount of sessions is based more on the client's uniqueness rather than a predictable system.

At the beginning of my manual therapy career—when my reductionist understanding was that of musculoskeletal levers and pulleys—I would venture predictions. That all changed when my caseload grew in complexity, making my estimations frustratingly useless. Further, understanding the crucial role of the client as an active part of the healing process made me realize how pointless, and borderline irresponsible, it was to predict a number of sessions without first starting treatment. Thus, whenever prospective clients ask: "*How many sessions will it take?*" I respond with: "*I won't know until I start treatment.*"

Age plays a significant role. Older clients are more likely to have carried pain and dysfunctions much longer than their younger counterparts, thus, the more compensatory patterns or layers they will harbor, thus necessitating more sessions. Then there's the client's involvement. In general, those who take care of their wellness respond better to treatment and need fewer sessions.

Then there are those who experienced evident injury or an acute pain episode likely driven by a microinjury. I make sure they understand that inflammation is a normal part of healing and as long as their tissues are healing, they will be producing more inflammation than usual and may need more continuous follow-up visits.

Also, there are those whose goals are to incorporate Counterstrain as a component of a healthier lifestyle. Personally, a preventive session once a month has done wonders for my health and wellness. Athletes and highly active individuals usually get treatment every four to six weeks as preventive medicine and to enhance performance. There are also those with long-term conditions who find that periodic Counterstrain treatment enhances the quality of their lives. Finally, there's work I considered sacred and it's for those with terminal conditions who receive Counterstrain to ease their suffering as they prepare to transition.

It is important to point out that there's a confounding factor that throws off any predictions in the number of sessions, and it is the client's default perceptual state. Those whose sympathetic nervous systems (SNS) are in chronic activation whether from life circumstances such as work, family, etc., or established behaviors such as type A personalities, control issues, anger, depression, etc., or when attention is highjacked by polarized news, rage-baiting content, etc., create a physiological environment that's not conducive to healing but prone to relapsing. We've analyzed the effects of the SNS enough to understand why.

For my practice, all I can do is recommend a number of follow-up sessions based on my findings. Because of the complexity of my caseload, the likelihood of solving it all in one session is virtually nonexistent, but I'll admit that there have been instances in which clients recovered fully after only one session or two. Those are exceptions and not representative of the majority.

I'll close this by stating that if I ever figure out the formula to produce recovery in a linear and certain basis—and without your intervention—then I'll charge ten times my rate and allow you to say: "*Fix me!*" Truth is, no one can. There are many factors involved in recovery and most of them are within the client's control.

Mixing Counterstrain with Other Modalities

The client would feel amazing and pain-free after her Counterstrain sessions. Alas, she would return the week after, in pain and frustrated. That was my head-scratcher in the summer of 2013 as I couldn't figure out why the carryover was so short-lived. But the answer was revealed when she arrived late for one of her sessions.

She was in a frantic state and requested to finish fifteen minutes earlier. When I asked if everything was okay she mentioned that she had made scheduling mistakes, and not only had her preceding physical therapy session run late, but only then did she realize that her chiropractic session overlapped with ours and she didn't want to be late. In addition, she had scheduled massage after chiropractic. I asked why she had booked all those sessions on the same day and she replied that she was being strategic.

"I do this every week. The chiropractor works on the bones, physical therapy strengthens the muscles, massage relaxes the muscles, and you ..." She looked at me, her hand searching the air. "Well, I don't know what you work on, but I feel really good after," she said.

I understood, then, that there was too much work on the same body. Though the rationale of inflammatory stasis wouldn't surface for another eight years, I knew how powerful the effects of Counterstrain were, and how much energy the body demanded for recovery after the sessions.

I am grateful that this happened early in my career. It provided me with context to notice incidents like this, which are more frequent than I could've imagined. Many emergency calls are the result of clients getting aggressive therapy shortly after Counterstrain, or from work done by therapists who presumed to understand Counterstrain but in reality didn't.

For clients who ask about combining modalities, I direct them to get them no fewer than two days prior their Counterstrain session, and no fewer than five to seven days after, depending on the complexity of their case. For those insisting on combining modalities the same day, I ask to be removed from the equation until their other therapies have completed their cycles.

Are there exceptions? Absolutely! I have productive relationships with practitioners of other modalities, and combining our work—even in the same day—has benefited the client. The difference is that these practitioners are well acquainted with Counterstrain, not only in its physiological rationale and principles, but also as clients who receive regular treatment. In addition, there are many high-level Counterstrain therapists who also practice other modalities and won't hesitate to combine them as needed. Ultimately, though, the client is in charge and they're free to choose if, or how, or when to combine modalities.

I am a big fan of all healing arts and I use them at different times or circumstances. All of them—including Counterstrain—have their specific effects in our bodies, which we have to understand if we are to combine them. In fact, the rebalancing process after Counterstrain therapy has its own quirks, and that's what we're going to explore next.

HOW WILL I FEEL AFTER A COUNTERSTRAIN SESSION?

The evolution of Counterstrain has turned it into one of the ultimate approaches for acute and chronic pain, and also for systemic and idiopathic conditions. This evolution also improved how the body processes its post-treatment changes. Though the application of Fascial Counterstrain has always been gentle, the same could not be said of its post-treatment effects in some clients in the earlier years.

These clients experienced a form of post-treatment malaise that would last between one to two days before the body settled and allowed them to enjoy the benefits of their session. Every new client was warned of some possible post-treatment effects and that it was a normal part of the process.

Thanks to the understanding of interstitial inflammatory stasis, the evolution of the lymphatic/venous techniques, and the evolution of the diagnostics systems, the incidences of post-treatment malaise have been significantly reduced. That doesn't mean they are completely eliminated, though. It is theorized that one of the factors driving these post-treatment effects may be our bodies reacting to trapped proinflammatory mediators reentering circulation on their way to being expelled. The reactions might be similar as if one were experiencing an injury, infection, or substance which, depending on the client, may be barely noticeable or quite uncomfortable.

The other factors are fluid rebalancing and mechanical tension redistribution, which is a normal process after shutting off protective reflex arcs that created unnecessary tissue tension and fluid entrapment. How the body rebalances its fluids and redistributes tensegrity is dependent on multiple factors, most outside the therapist's control, or the client's voluntary control.

It's hard to predict with certainty who might experience post-treatment effects or what type of effects. Releasing trapped inflammation does not produce a single sensation but a spectrum of reactions that vary widely from person to person as the trapped inflammation is channeled for elimination. Some of the most common are:

- Sleepiness
- Lethargy
- Soreness
- Occasionally, some may experience:
- Chills
- Hot flashes
- Minor headaches
- Sadness
- Euphoria
- Moodiness

There may be a few more, but at this point the more important question is, *Will you be one of those who experience post-treatment effects?* Experience has shown me that the factors that influence your number of sessions will also influence how you'll feel after treatment. For instance:

- **Your Medical History.** In general, those with a history of systemic conditions (MS, Lyme disease, Crohn's, celiac, severe allergies, etc.), intensive treatments (chemotherapy, radiation, large doses of antibiotics, etc.), multiple surgeries, or multiple traumas, tend to experience the most post-treatment effects. It is not uncommon for clients with a history of severe infections to experience a Jarisch-Herxheimer, or Herx, reaction, possibly due to trapped particles from dead pathogens and/or their endotoxins reentering circulation before being expelled. In addition, clients with a history of concussions, craniofacial injuries, craniofacial surgeries, or intensive dental work may be more susceptible due to the proximity to the CNS.

- **Length of the dysfunction.** In general, the longer you've been harboring the dysfunction, the greater the chances you'll experience some post-treatment effects. Keep in mind that the time you experienced symptoms is not necessarily the time you've harbored the dysfunction.

- **Age.** In general, the older you are, the greater the number of dysfunctions you may have, thus, the greater the likelihood you'll experience post-treatment effects.

- **Experience.** Those who receive Counterstrain on a maintenance basis rarely experience post-treatment effects, and if they do, they're mild. This seems to wear off, though, if the client goes six months or longer without treatment.

- **Physical Fitness.** My most reliable predictor and the big equalizer. Physically fit individuals fare the best, regardless of age or other factors. They rarely experience post-treatment effects, and if they do, it's short-lived. It's an excellent reason to emphasize productive strength training and fitness in our lives.

What to Do?

While the discomfort dissipates in twenty-four to forty-eight hours for most, there are a few tried-and-true methods to help you ease the process:

- **Hydrate.** All that trapped inflammation will be eventually peed away, so staying hydrated will optimize the process.
- **Sleep.** Get a full night rest, and if you need more, take a couple of short naps during the day.
- **Warm Showers.** Even more helpful prior to bed.
- **Epsom Salt Baths.** Enough said! Enjoy.
- **Arnica.** Popular in homeopathic medicine, it can be used in gel, oil, or pellet form. Make sure to consult with your physician first.
- **Leisurely Stroll.** A gentle walk in the fresh air can help you clear your head and body.

Your therapist will have a better idea of how you might react only after your session, so please pay attention to their recommendations. Keep in mind that this doesn't happen to everyone but you may still get the heads-up as a precaution. Overall, this will be a great time to embrace patience and respect your body. After all, it's only letting you know that you need to rest so it can continue the healing process.

THE ART IN FCS THERAPY: CONNECTING TO THE HUMAN

At this point, you've become familiar with the components of the FCS experience and why its results are so remarkable. We, as practitioners, get to repeatedly witness its immense power and though our clients are happy to give us testimonials, they're also hesitant about sharing the details of their cases. All perfectly understandable.

In these days where testimonials and reviews can be easily purchased or stolen, it's difficult to discern what's legit and what's not. The same cannot be said of case studies, where the details can be traced and confirmed. However, presenting a case study in a manner that appeals to the general public and also the scientific community is a gigantic task only a few are willing to undertake. Fortunately, Brian Tuckey did this as part of his methodology article with the case of a nurse practitioner whose life was altered by failed medical interventions [26]. You can access all the details—including some of the treatments and their descriptions—as well as videos of the initial conditions and treatment progress by using the QR code or link below.

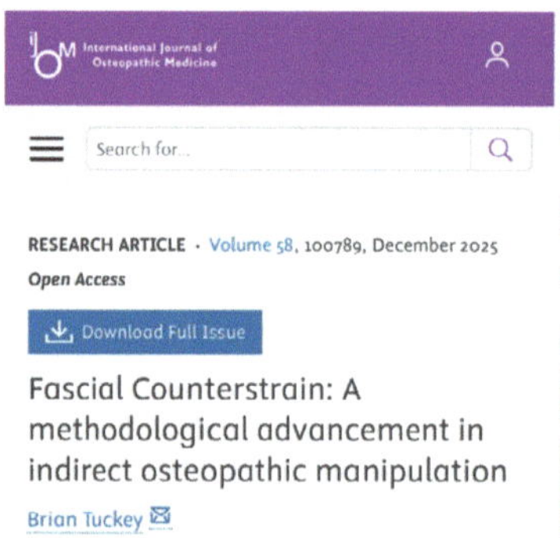
International Journal of Osteopathic Medicine

Search for...

RESEARCH ARTICLE · Volume 58, 100789, December 2025

Open Access

Download Full Issue

Fascial Counterstrain: A methodological advancement in indirect osteopathic manipulation

Brian Tuckey

journalofosteopathicmedicine.com/article/S1746-0689(25)00045-8/fulltext

Her case is remarkable in two aspects. One, it highlights the efficacy of FCS in resolving what seems impossible. And two, this case connect us with the humanity of the client—the element that merges all our governing principles into an art form. We can talk about releasing IIS, its effects on our physiology, or central sensitization, but the art of treatment requires connecting with our clients and acknowledging their sentience and struggles.

One of our core credos is that *Counterstrain changes lives, not just symptoms*. The brightness in the eyes, the smile, and the gratitude that follow the resolution of a complex case reward the thousands of hours of practice, learning, and the sacrifices that cultivating our skills demands. I'm certain that this case will inspire you as much as it inspired me. More than a testament to our therapeutic system, it is a reminder that the ultimate result is returning the joy of life to a soul that had lost hope.

Where do We Go from Here?

There is no going back, that much I can tell you with absolute certainty. Brian Tuckey had already arrived at the governing principles of Fascial Counterstrain in the early 2000s, but the relevant research to sustain his hypothesis was still years behind. He understood that for the emerging field of Fascial Counterstrain to get the attention of the scientific community, he had to have quality peer-reviewed material to support his discoveries.

Just so you understand how far ahead Brian was, the crucial study conducted by Dr. Jay P. Shah—in which he discovered elevated proinflammatory markers in trigger points—was published in January 2008. That means the process started much earlier, likely in 2006. And this didn't happen on a whim. Dr. Shah was a client of Brian's, and as a National Institute of Health (NIH) researcher and clinician he wanted to know what in the world Brian was doing that made such a difference in his chronic pain [14]. It was then that Brian presented his hypothesis, which was then presented to the NIH, where it gathered sufficient attention to allow Dr. Shah to conduct the pertinent work.

Nowadays, thanks to advances in medical technology, relevant studies continue bringing light to what Brian knew all along and to what we experience on our treatment tables on a daily basis. Yet it's still not enough. Many dismiss the novel theoretical rationale as a mere educated guess because it has yet to be researched under different environments.

But history shows us that many of our modern proven scientific principles were at first novel theories dismissed as ho-hum because they still had to gather more evidence. Take the germ theory of disease, which was considered superstition until Pasteur, Koch, and other scientists proved it with experiments in the nineteenth century. Our modern times feature other examples. Take neuroplasticity, which challenged the notion that the adult brain was fixed and immutable. Neuroplasticity theories were confronted until clinical cases and advanced imaging studies proved how the brain is capable of regenerating itself even after what could be considered a devastating brain injury.

Now take a look at the flowchart of physiological interactions driving IIS and the subsequent self-perpetuating loop of pain, dysfunction, and tissue damage.

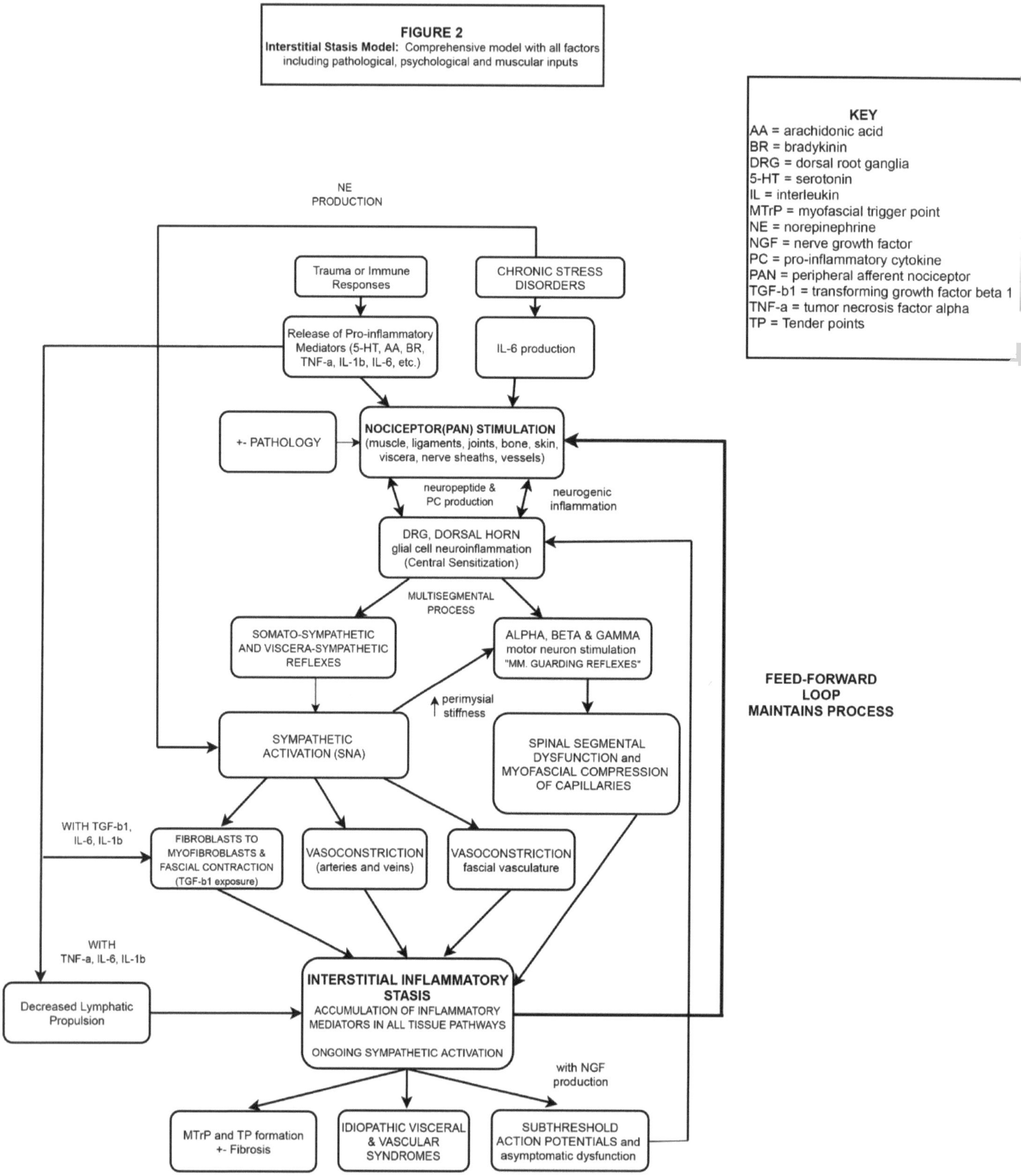

Figure 2 from the August 22, 2021, Impaired Lymphatic Drainage article published in Frontiers in Pain Research. Flowchart reproduced with permission of Brian Tuckey.

All the components—which we reviewed in the previous pages—are scientifically documented. Trapped inflammation [35], the existence of interstitium and microvasculature [32], central sensitization [43], the effects of chronic sympathetic nervous system activation [58], the formation of fibrosis and tissue degeneration from cytokine exposure [54], muscle guarding reflexes [45], and the existence and significance of trigger points/tender points—all are well documented and have also been confirmed by diagnostic ultrasound [85].

Remember that all those components are the results of meticulous research and testing in their own specific niche, thus, they all exist exclusively in their own specific niche, and rarely do researchers look beyond their own niche. It was Brian who stepped outside the confines of conventional manual therapy and pored over the literature from diverse branches of pain research to put the pieces together. The role of science is to observe and measure probabilities, not define absolutes, and as a result, researchers investigating the nature of complex pain are looking at his hypothesis as a key component of their research puzzles and citing his article in their publications [86] [87].

I've been told that the remarkable FCS results could be a placebo effect driven by hope and heightened expectations. While that's a possibility, it doesn't explain the dozens of skeptics who were convinced there was nothing I could do to help them, only to become ardent fans once they experienced the results. Heck, I'm sometimes skeptical myself. I recently saw a client with severe neck issues that were the result of multiple traumas. Her cervical spine images resembled a Jenga puzzle and she had not responded to any modalities. Both of us were skeptical about any resolution, more so when her allodynia demanded significant treatment modifications. To both our surprises, she reported remarkable reduction in pain, discomfort, and stiffness after twenty-four hours, and being able to sleep through the night for the first time in years. Rarely, though, are such case reports considered valuable when compiling data.

Those of us who have embraced Counterstrain as our calling are well acquainted with the complexities of all the physiological interactions governing our modality. We acknowledge the demands that FCS mastery requires: superb multidimensional anatomical knowledge, superb touch and palpatory skills, unencumbered kinesthetic awareness that makes the flow of Counterstrain possible, and the ability to deliver treatment with finesse and precision.

None of us arrived in the field with those traits but were willing to make the necessary investments to acquire them. Thousands of hours of supervised training, practice, studying, and frustration, as well as a significant investment of resources—all were a worthy price for such skills. Being able to find those concealed pools of inflammation and releasing them with no discomfort is a feeling that transcends words. It's magical and scientific at the same time, technical yet unpredictable, fluid as a dance where expert dancers perfectly synchronize with the music. Seeing our clients' eyes reclaim the volume and glimmer of health is an immense reward.

I often reflect on how I would not have been able to help so many clients, or fulfill my mission, had I not followed the unorthodox path that led me to Counterstrain. As I just mentioned, even with all my experience I still harbor doubts when some wild cases walk into my practice. But Counterstrain continues guiding me. As long as I honor its principles, I find the path in the majority of those convoluted cases. And yes, there are times when no matter what I do, I make no difference. I'm human after all, but it's those failures that drive me to keep learning.

I am excited for the future of the field. The advances in treatment and rationale have weeded out those who only looked at Counterstrain casually but have attracted those who desire nothing less than life-transforming mastery. Also, the advent of the Counterstrain Convention, thanks to the efforts of the Counterstrain Academy, has made it possible for Counterstrain practitioners of all levels to experience an environment of immersion, guidance, and interaction that is virtually impossible in other settings. Our skills always skyrocket right after these conventions.

I am excited for the future of Counterstrain because the number of qualified and proficient practitioners grows every year. More and more people are discovering the power of Counterstrain, and we are starting to emerge from the shadows of anonymity. It's only a matter of time before the term Counterstrain becomes akin to hope. All of my colleagues are on similar journeys and all of us are eager to welcome you as a client or as colleague.

How do I Find a Counterstrain Therapist?

Up until a few years ago that was a question that would make me uncomfortable. It came from clients who simply wanted to know where their friends and family in other corners of the world could experience the power of FCS. It would make me uncomfortable because I didn't have a solid answer. Back then, there was only a handful of us and even fewer at the advanced levels.

That's no longer the case. The evolution of our field has attracted excellent candidates and has also made skill acquisition more streamlined, but it still takes time and dedicated practice to turn an eager novice into a proficient, safe, and effective FCS therapist. Though this extensive training makes our growth slow, it also makes it sustainable. Our numbers may still be small compared to other modalities, with the bulk of therapists located in the continental US, but there are more of us nonetheless.

The internet is our ally and since you're reading this, I'll assume you're looking for qualified practitioners dedicated to mastery. In that case, there are only two websites you should explore.

The first website is that of the Counterstrain Academy (**counterstrain.com**) and the second one is that of the Jones Institute website (**jicounterstrain.com**). Both have searchable directories to help you locate a Counterstrain therapist by zip code or city.

The difference is that the Counterstrain Academy lists only practitioners who have completed at least four modules, whereas the Jones Institute lists all of their students. I'll give you more detailed info on the resources page.

The rest is up to you. All of us share the same passion and do everything in our power to be the best therapists we can be, but we all run our practices differently. All of us have our policies and rates accessible, as well as our availability, but we are all different in how we book, take payments, and communicate. It is up to you to figure out which you find more agreeable.

This is now the point where you use this book to prepare you for your session. Refer to the pertinent sections if you feel tempted to ask your therapist whether they can help you with your issue (they *won't* know until they assess you) how many sessions it will take (they WON'T know until they asses you) or if they know what caused it (they *won't* know until they assess you).

You also have to be honest with yourself and your condition. If all you have is minor aches and pains, or if you're in good health and need some basic maintenance, any practitioner with a couple of modules should suffice. However, if you're dealing with systemic conditions, or have a history of concussions, multiple traumas, and/or surgeries, you'll need the most advanced therapist you can find.

One of the aspects I appreciate about our community is how most practitioners are cognizant of their limitations and won't hesitate to refer to advanced therapists when needed. Provided that you're being proactive in your own healing, your encounter with Counterstrain will be revealing and pleasant.

HOW DO I BECOME A COUNTERSTRAIN THERAPIST?

Earlier on, I said that the most soul-crushing feeling for a therapist is the inability to help our clients despite our best efforts. This frustration eventually leads to burning out and quitting the field.

That's what I was experiencing until Counterstrain helped me regain my fire, my sanity, and transformed my practice. There can be long days and puzzling days, but never, *ever*, a boring day, or a day in which I don't learn something. My soul rejoices whenever I recognize that I'm not only fulfilling my mission, I'm also part of a movement that's permanently reshaping how we heal our bodies.

Now, if your therapist heart feels lighter and energized at the potential of Counterstrain, then you may have what it takes to be part of our community. We come from different backgrounds but we all share commonalities. We take it personally when we see others suffering from pain and get consumed with finding ways to relieve that pain. We have all experienced or witnessed how the gentle application of Counterstrain brought resolution to what others considered dead ends. We are all humbled and inspired by this magnificent approach and are obsessed with learning and practicing simply because we want to continue improving. But our greatest strength is our ability to let go—to unlearn, if you will—of what we had once embraced, even though we had copiously invested time and resources to learn it.

There's no other way. Letting go of the conventional is what creates the room to absorb and embody the essence of the governing FCS principles. You may learn the techniques, but applying the techniques without honoring the principles will result in more frustration than success. Letting go may be uncomfortable, but it's satisfying.

Ultimately, your work will pay off as you acquire jaw-dropping skills that solve the most unusual problems gently, effectively, and quickly. Your clients will be convinced that what you practice is a miracle and you won't be able to convince them otherwise.

Are you ready?

First Things First!

You must be a licensed professional in a relevant healthcare field. This includes:

- Physical therapists
- Occupational therapists
- Massage therapists
- Chiropractors
- Orthopedists
- Osteopaths
- Naturopaths
- MDs
- Acupuncturists

As to which field will give you the best advantage, none of them really will. Counterstrain training is the big equalizer and depending on your field, you'll realize that where some therapists of different backgrounds struggle, you'll succeed with ease. The reverse will also be true. Be prepared to get out of your comfort zone.

Next

Go to the **Jones Institute** website to register for the **Foundations of Fascial Counterstrain** course. This initial step is mandatory for every student regardless of their background. You will not be allowed to register for other courses without the Foundations class.

Then practice what you have learned. Keep practicing and then continue practicing until the principles and their applications feel less awkward. The Jones Institute now provides all novice students with an excellent online platform to preview and review the most salient aspects of the Foundations course. Once you feel confident in your basic skills, register for your next course. I highly recommend the lymphatic/venous modules as the follow-up to Foundations.

Then practice! Practice until the principles and therapeutic approaches are part of you. This is the point at which the casual onlookers throw in the towel. Practice is the simplest but most demanding component of mastery. Once you feel confident in your mastery of the new material, take the next course. Then, practice, practice, and practice some more until the new material is second nature and integrated with the previous material. Rinse and repeat.

Not a day goes by in which I don't look back at those intense days of practice without immense gratitude. They were demanding but also immeasurably rewarding and a lot of fun. It was as if I was being transported to a different dimension, where the pleasure of learning and discovery are so immense that linear time ceases and our stamina perpetuates. It is what keeps all proficient therapists in this journey, and I hope that one day you also get to experience it.

It is too Much!

"There are two types of people; those who don't know how to improve, and those who don't know when to stop."

CHRIS WILLIAMSON

We have all been there. The point at which it feels like no matter how hard we try; we can't figure things out. The point where no matter how much we practice, we still fail. The point that no matter how much we study, we can't grasp what we study anymore.

You're not alone. No proficient therapist has achieved mastery without experiencing those frustrations. While we will never be immune to them, we've been in the game long enough to learn to take full advantage of all the available resources to help us overcome that funk. Here are a few to help both novice and seasoned therapists.

- **Download and register for the Counterstrain 3D app.** The app is a fantastic reference for you and your clients, with a clear location of the relevant tender points and a description of the pertinent techniques. This app is activated only for the courses you've taken. While you may be able to download it without taking a course, you won't be able to use it. There's a verification process all of us must follow before given access to requested modules. The advantage of the app is that it can be easily accessed from any mobile device as well as desktops, and we can have immediate access to refinements and updates.
- **Take the course again.** I love how the established Counterstrain courses get constantly refined and updated. I retake each course every two or three years, and while it will feel familiar, it will also feel brand-new. There have been so many *a-ha!* moments and so many gems I received while retaking the courses that it's my favorite strategy to overcome overwhelm and doubt. Besides, the Jones Institute offers a discount for retaking any course. Win-win!
- **Take a module with the Counterstrain Academy.** Sometimes the depth of the material presented during the typical weekend course could feel overwhelming. Some would like more time to review the concepts, more personalized attention, or more practice time. This is where the Counterstrain Academy comes in. They cover the material in more depth over a couple of weekends instead of one. The classes are smaller for more personalized attention, and you get to meet other passionate practitioners.

- **Attend the Counterstrain Convention.** This amazing and energetic event held every two or three years is open to all students who have completed at least the Foundations course. The first one took place in August 2018 and marked an important step in the evolution of Counterstrain education. Since then, the convention has been the perfect vehicle to deliver updates, research breakthroughs, and refinements in an environment that cannot be replicated in a typical classroom setting. It is also an amazing opportunity to practice and mingle with Counterstrain therapists from all over the country and all over the world.

But ... *What if all fails? What if after all of it, the overwhelm lingers?*

I believe that passionate and dedicated practice is the foundation of mastery and nothing will ever substitute it. But even dedicated practice has its limits. We are all human and we will all eventually reach a point where, no matter what we do, we can absorb no more. At this point—as counterproductive as it may seem—the best strategy is to take a break and let our minds get much-needed rest to process the lessons. Experience has shown me that we won't forget what we've learned. In fact, after a couple of weeks away from dedicated practice, my understanding comes together on its own and brings new revelations, thus revamping my energy and getting me ready to learn even more.

Know that you will never be alone and that you can always reach out to the Counterstrain community with your concerns. Our social media groups are dynamic and we are always looking out for each other. We look forward to welcoming you as a colleague and to the life-changing journey of Counterstrain mastery.

SELF-EVIDENT AND UNDENIABLE

History is full of brilliant health professionals who explored the unconventional when the established protocols failed them. Andrew T. Still, William G. Sutherland, and John E. Upledger, among others, caused controversy when their visions defied the norms [74]. It wasn't peer-reviewed research that led these healers to break from convention—it was their intuition.

Our intuition is far more powerful than we could possibly imagine, but we choke it off when we believe we need permission from conventional protocols before embarking on exploration. The aforementioned healers are the perfect example of what happens when an open mind and intuition defy what others consider infallible.

The late Dr. Jones also comes to mind, as does Brian Tuckey. It was Dr. Jones' intuition that first guided him to explore what many would've dismissed as a coincidence, and it was Brian's intuition what led him to recognize that Dr. Jones' work affected far more than what was considered possible. Dr. Jones had confided to Brian that his biggest concern was that Counterstrain would disappear after his passing. Brian promised him then that he would not allow that to happen, and he's kept his word. As the modern version of Counterstrain continues evolving and word of mouth about its effectiveness spreads, health professionals and the general public want to learn more. And those are the people for whom I wrote this book.

And I also wrote it to honor those whose lives were changed by this modality. Although they can sense its application and effectiveness, and even understand the physiological principles for themselves, they still have a hard time communicating the experience to their loved ones without sounding crazy. This is for you and them.

But I also wrote this because prospective clients show up to our practices with false expectations driven by misinformation, and because the still-prevalent misconceptions about our bodies can interfere, even negate, the results of the treatment. I have too much respect for the dedication put forth by the minds improving the system to just let this slip by.

I didn't write this to convince anyone to try Counterstrain or pursue it as a career, as I did. The virtues of the modality were self-evident and undeniable, and it was only my desire to improve as a therapist, healer, and health professional that fueled my efforts.

It was not an easy path. I started my Counterstrain journey during a difficult period in my life. Late 2010 had seen the dissolution of my business venture. Whatever funds I had were spent on bringing closure to the old and starting the new.

If you were to ask me how I afforded my Counterstrain training, I would not be able to tell you. All I know is that I invested funds that I didn't have then, but I knew I'd recoup them. All the Counterstrain classes and mastery modules that I've taken have repaid that investment many times over. I don't know with linear certainty how, but I know in my heart that not having Counterstrain in my life would be far costlier.

Practitioners from other modalities have told me that Counterstrain is not the only system to help people with their pain and dysfunction, and I agree one hundred percent. Day in and day out, countless practitioners in many modalities are helping their clients regain their active lifestyle and joy of living.

Counterstrain may not be the only system to help those in pain, but in my experience, it's the only one dramatically reshaping how we approach manual therapy medicine. I'll go as far as saying that while our principles are sound science, the treatment itself is an art form in which we engage all of our senses as we interact with our clients, and such an ability demands committed practice and continuous learning.

Yet I keep an open mind for other approaches that could revolutionize my practice as FCS did. If there's another indirect system that can outperform its success rate in cases considered hopeless, and can do so gently and efficiently, then the circumstances that guided me to Counterstrain will guide me there. In my experience, those claiming to match Counterstrain did not understand it or were clinging to outdated therapeutic models and biases.

Dr. Jones' legacy lives on as Brian Tuckey relentlessly continues researching and challenging the notions of what's possible. What an amazing time to be a Counterstrain therapist.

Wishing you a joyous, energized, and pain-free life.
COACH IZZY

COUNTERSTRAIN RESOURCES

Counterstrain has grown in depth, reach, and presence since my first class in April 2012. It may not yet be a dominant modality, but it's not a mystery either. The days of scarce and inconsistent resources are long gone, and finding valuable, updated, and more accurate information is easier.

Whether you are a therapist who is frustrated with the lack of progress of their clients, or a prospective client frustrated with the lack of progress or answers, the resources in this page should guide you to the right place.

The Jones Institute

Founded in 1988 by Dr. Jones himself and Randall "Randy" Kusunose, PT, OCS, JSCCI, it is the destination for licensed healthcare professionals eager to explore and learn the science of Counterstrain. Randy is credited with taking Counterstrain from a realm that was exclusive to osteopaths to a broader range of licensed healthcare practitioners.

You can go to their website, **jicounterstrain.com,** and explore some of the options described next.

> **Counterstrain Training.** The Jones Institute is the official educational organization offering training in Strain-Counterstrain and Fascial Counterstrain, and it does so through a rich curriculum. From your first steps into the modality all the way to central sensitization treatment, the flow is designed to maximize your skill development and proficiency. Fascial Counterstrain classes are hosted at the Jones Institute and its many satellites across the country. For those desiring to explore Dr. Jones' legacy work as it was developed, Strain-Counterstrain training is still offered exclusively at the Jones Institute.
>
> **Brain Dissection.** This incredible resource is open to all licensed healthcare practitioners, not just Counterstrain therapists, though you will find them in significant attendance. This dynamic three-day, hands-on experience explores brain structure, function, and pathologies via dissection and targeted lectures. A must for all those seeking to understand more about perceptual dysregulation disorders, neuroinflammation, and central sensitization.

Pelvic Floor Dissection. Another excellent educational resource that is open to all licensed healthcare practitioners. This two-day course allows students the opportunity to dissect and identify the anatomy of the pelvis, and explore the structures that make up the pelvic diaphragm and the neurovascular structures involved in its function. There is emphasis on exploring the structural and physiological differences between male and female anatomy as well as their functional role on micturition, elimination, and sexual function.

Unembalmed Cadaver Dissection. This five-day, 30-hour course is open to all licensed healthcare practitioners and it's one of my favorites because—unlike most dissection courses—we work with unembalmed bodies. This allows us to interact with our systems and structures in a way that's impossible with embalmed donors. It's a sacred and powerful experience with emphasis on exploring neural networks, blood supply, and drainage. One can easily identify and dissect over 1,000 anatomical structures and get a more in-depth understanding of their functions, clinical relevance, and role in pathologies. As a bonus, the pelvic floor dissection course is included. Not to be missed.

Practitioner Directory. Whether you have taken one class or the entire curriculum, the Jones Institute offers you the option to be part of their directory. Your selected contact information as well as your Counterstrain trainings and certifications will be visible to those searching the directory for a practitioner.

The Jones Institute YouTube Channel. This channel is a treasure of information that will help you cement your understanding of Counterstrain and will keep you up to date about their educational resources. I highly recommend the discussions between Kyle Kusunose and Brian Tuckey as they go, in depth, over the effects of IIS, the ensuing pathologies, and how Fascial Counterstrain addresses them. A must for those seeking to improve their understanding of our field. The link is **youtube.com/channel/UC7oLJFs7wCp81gn2KTes0JA**

I couldn't conclude without emphasizing that there are only two institutions authorized to teach and train Counterstrain methods. Though some would claim otherwise, unless the CEC certificate comes from either the Jones Institute or the Counterstrain Academy, it is a modality that's anything but actual Counterstrain.

The Counterstrain Academy

The Counterstrain Academy was founded by Timothy Hodges in 2005 when therapists struggling with the science and skills specific to Counterstrain sought his expertise and guidance. What started as a handful of students evolved to become the Counterstrain Academy, currently located in Portland, Oregon. The academy is the only Counterstrain mastery program of its kind and is responsible for helping hundreds of aspiring therapists deepen their understanding and sharpen their skills.

The focus of the Academy is the development of Fascial Counterstrain, and its contributions cement this vision. In addition to developing unique learning resources, it also established Counterstrain and its logo as an official international trademark in the fall of 2017. These efforts have helped protect and preserve the legacy of Dr. Jones and launched Counterstrain as an upcoming force.

Though the Counterstrain Academy and the Jones Institute operate independently from each other, they work in cohesion for the greatest benefit of all students. Aspiring therapists and potential clients visit **counterstrain.com** to explore in-depth training opportunities and to find therapists committed to mastery.

> **In-Depth Review of Counterstrain Modules.** There are two essential requirements to attend the Academy's mastery modules. One, you have to be a licensed healthcare professional. Two, whatever module you want to pursue with the Academy, you must have already taken it with the Jones Institute. There's no way around those requirements and the Academy has a verification process.
>
> Tim Hodges created the program at the request of practitioners who felt overwhelmed by the amount of complex information in the three-day classes. They needed more personalized attention, a more digestible pace, and wanted to take their skills to a higher level. The mastery program provided them all. Classes are spread out over two weekends instead of one, with small groups that allow ample time for questions, review, and practice.
>
> I credit the Counterstrain Academy mastery program with transforming this eager novice into an effective and proficient practitioner in barely over a year. I highly encourage all practitioners to take at least a couple of modules and notice the substantial improvements. Mastery classes are currently hosted at the Portland headquarters and some international destinations.

3D Counterstrain App. Counterstrain technique charts were our best allies when Jones' Strain-Counterstrain was the primary form of our modality. Whether on office walls or on clipboards, the charts proved an invaluable reference resource. Alas, practical as they were for Strain-Counterstrain, they were not ideal for the constant updates and developments of the fascial model.

That's when Brian Tuckey and Tim Hodges pooled their resources to commission an interactive app dedicated to Fascial Counterstrain. This app allows therapists to review tender points and their techniques from a high-resolution, 3D model, and to receive updates to the curriculum. The app is available for mobile devices and tablets running iOS or Android operating systems and can also be accessed via laptop or desktop. While you can download it from your mobile app store, you won't be able to purchase or have access to the modules until the Academy verifies your status.

The Counterstrain Convention. August 2018 marked an important step in the evolution of the Counterstrain Academy with the introduction of the first Counterstrain Convention. This five-day educational event is held every two or three years and it's open to experienced and novice practitioners who have completed at the least the Foundations course. It is also a great opportunity to meet and mingle from practitioners from all over the country and all over the world.

The experience provides an environment of immersion in selected modules and offers ample guidance and help from instructors. You will also be exposed to the latest updates and research breakthroughs, usually well ahead of the rest of the community. Besides being an excellent opportunity to immerse in established modules, the convention is also the perfect vehicle to deliver supplemental modules.

Supplemental Modules. The enormous advancement of Fascial Counterstrain also meant the advancement of its modules, which also expanded the power of our modality but also increased class content. For some modules, the expansions required the material to be split into two classes to maximize their potential.

But for a few other modules the expanded material presented a conundrum. If added to the regular classes it would choke an already packed syllabus, but it wasn't sufficient on its own to warrant another three-day class. That's when the Counterstrain Academy introduced one-day supplemental module trainings at the conventions. Thanks to these supplemental modules, many practitioners were able to expand the power of their work by adding techniques for epidural ligaments and vasculature, specific spinal periosteal work, tendon vasculature, and more. As with the regular Counterstrain Academy modules, participants must have already taken the corresponding three-day class.

Practitioner Directory. The Counterstrain Academy website also has a searchable practitioner directory. The main difference between theirs and the Jones Institute directory is that practitioners wishing to be listed in the Academy site must have completed at least four of the regular Fascial Counterstrain modules, which the Academy will verify. Information about all the modules you've completed with the Jones Institute and the Academy, certification status, as well as your bio and a link to your practice are available to those who qualify for this directory.

Tuckey and Associates Clinic

Information about Brian Tuckey's clinic, Fascial Counterstrain, and Counterstrain Training. Brian's practice is one of the busiest in the country, and though he may not see you directly as he oversees only the most complex cases, his staff is highly trained and more than qualified to also tackle complex cases.

For those seeking FCS training, visiting his clinic for a few classes is a worthwhile experience as you may get input directly from Brian himself. Their website is **tuckeypt.com**

The Counterstrain Movement Podcast

Why is it that after all these years of mind-blowing results. so many people still haven't heard about FCS? There are many reasons but the most prevalent is that the developers and high-level practitioners dedicate most of their time and resources to honing their craft and running their busy practices.

Spreading the word in popular media demands additional time and resources that the busy practitioner may not feel like undertaking, lest they burn out. But we all know it's necessary and luckily, technology is making this task easier.

Enter one of the latest efforts to make FCS known to the general public, **The Counterstrain Movement Podcast**, an online production dedicated to exploring the origins of Counterstrain, its mechanics, the conditions it treats, and how you can incorporate it in your life. Features in-depth interviews with instructors, therapists, and clients about the power of our modality. It's hosted by Theora Moench edited by Haley Diaz, and produced by **The Bridge Back Project**. You can enjoy it on your favorite online/mobile platform or go directly to **thecounterstrainmovement.buzzsprout.com**

The Bridge Back Project

This 501(c)3 organization founded by Dr. Holly Christy, ND, LAc, CACI, JSCCI, CSC I, is dedicated to bringing Fascial Counterstrain to address the impact of trauma, to promote healing, and to restore hope. It relies on your donations to make their three essential priorities tangible, so they can make high-quality FCS available to those dealing with the life-disrupting effects of trauma.

These three essential priorities—Accessibility, Education, and Research—have made it possible for our field to reach a broader audience, thanks to efforts like **The Counterstrain Movement** podcast, and to gain recognition as a science-based modality. Dr. Christy's work and research on FCS as an effective component in perceptual trauma healing was officially published in the August 2025 issue of the *Military Medicine Journal*, bringing light to the neurophysiology of trauma and helping change the way people understand, talk about, and treat trauma-impacted individuals. Visit **bridgeback.org** to learn more about their mission and to contribute to its advancement.

REFERENCES

[1] L. H. Jones, "History of Counterstrain with founder Dr. Lawrence Jones," The Jones Institute YouTube Channel, 27 July 2020. [Online]. Available: https://youtu.be/K3CKBnIs6GI?si=DjF660qJLpyPuzWn.

[2] L. H. Jones, R. Kusunose and E. Goering, Jones Strain-Counterstrain, Boise, ID: Jones Strain-Counterstrain, Inc., 1995.

[3] I. M. Korr, "Proprioceptors and somatic dysfunction," *The Journal of the American Osteopathic Association,* pp. 638-650, 1975.

[4] R. L. Van Buskirk, "Nociceptive reflexes and the somatic dysfunction: A model," *Journal of Osteopathic Medicine,* vol. 90, no. 9, pp. 792 – 809, 1990.

[5] T. Hodges, *Counterstrain Convention Manual,* Portland, OR: Counterstrain Academy, 2021.

[6] M. C. Jensen, M. N. Brant-Zawadzki, N. Obuchowski, M. T. Modic, D. Malkasian and J. S. Ross, "Magnetic Resonance Imaging of the Lumbar Spine in People without Back Pain," *The New England Journal of Medicine,* vol. 331, no. 2, pp. 69-73, 1994.

[7] W. Brinjikji, P. H. Luetmer, B. Comstock, B. W. Bresnahan, L. E. Chen, R. A. Deyo, S. Halabi, J. A. Turner, A. L. Avins, K. James, J. T. Wald, D. F. Kallmes and J. G. Jarvik, "Systematic Literature Review of Imaging Features of Spinal Degeneration in Asymptomatic Populations," *AJNR American Journal of Neuroradiology,* vol. 36, no. 4, pp. 811 – 816, 2015.

[8] A. Ben-Yishay, "Axial Back Pain: Most Common Low Back Pain," Spine-health, 25 4 2012. [Online]. Available: https://www.spine-health.com/conditions/lower-back-pain/axial-back-pain-most-common-low-back-pain.

[9] N. Augeard and S. P. Carroll, "Core stability and low-back pain: a causal fallacy," *Journal of Exercise Rehabilitation,* vol. 15, no. 3, pp. 493-495, 2019.

[10] L. Mannix, "Is good posture overrated? Back to first principles on back pain," The Guardin, 5 August 2023. [Online]. Available: https://www.theguardian.com/science/2023/aug/06/good-posture-back-pain-how-to-avoid. [Accessed 2024].

[11] M. C. Siff, "Recommended Strength Ratios, Strength and Gender, Machine Testing?," in *Facts and Fallacies of Fitness,* Denver, CO, 2003, pp. 96, 153, 207-208.

[12] Lymphcast Podcast, Lymphcast Podcast, 30 August 2023. [Online]. Available: https://youtu.be/l3JgWedz4GE?feature=shared&t=2073.

[13] B. Tuckey, J. Srbely, G. Rigney, M. Vythilingam and J. Shah, "Impaired Lymphatic Drainage and Interstitial Inflammatory Stasis in Chronic Musculoskeletal and Idiopathic Pain Syndromes: a Novel Mechanism," *Frontiers in Pain Research,* vol. 2, 2021.

[14] K. Kusunose and B. Tuckey, "Spinal Ligament Dysfunctions You're Missing Without Counterstrain," The Jones Institute YouTube Channel, 15 January 2025. [Online]. Available: https://youtu.be/t3EJrA-KFLE?si=1q316AxfEr2Ya7KS.

[15] L. K. Koop and P. Tadi, "Neuroanatomy, Sensory Nerves," National Center for Biotechnology Information, 4 July 2023. [Online]. Available: https://www.ncbi.nlm.nih.gov/books/NBK539846/.

[16] M. P. Jankowski, K. K. Rau, K. M. Ekmann,, C. E. Anderson, and H. R. Koerber, "Comprehensive phenotyping of group III and IV muscle afferents in mouse," *Journal of Neurophysiology,* vol. 109, p. 2374 –2381, 2013.

[17] J. Bonar and M. Kumka, "Fascia: a morphological description and classification system based on a literature review," *The Journal of the Canadian Chiropractic Association,* vol. 56, no. 3, pp. 171 - 191, 2012.

[18] C. Wood, "Sending the Right Signals," BrainFacts.Org, 21 August 2017. [Online]. Available: https://www.brainfacts.org/brain-anatomy-and-function/cells-and-circuits/2017/image-of-the-week-sending-the-right-signals-082117.

[19] C. Cooley-Themm, "Interneurons | Definition, Function & Location," Study.com, 21 November 2023. [Online]. Available: https://study.com/learn/lesson/interneurons-function-diagram-location-association-neuron-example.html.

[20] M. Monte and W. C. Lloyd, "What are reflexes, and how do they work?," Medical News Today, 13 September 2023. [Online]. Available: https://www.medicalnewstoday.com/articles/what-are-reflexes.

[21] Q. Chen and M. M. Heinricher, "Shifting the Balance: How Top-Down and Bottom-Up Input Modulate Pain via the Rostral Ventromedial Medulla," *Frontiers in Pain Research,* vol. 3, pp. 1-9, 2022.

[22] Cleveland Clinic, "Cytokines," Cleveland Clinic, 3 January 2023. [Online]. Available: https://my.clevelandclinic.org/health/body/24585-cytokines.

[23] J.-M. Zhang and J. An, "Cytokines, Inflammation and Pain," *International Anesthesiology Clinics,* vol. 45, no. 2, pp. 27-37, 2007.

[24] C. Zanza, T. Romenskaya, A. C. Manetti, F. Franceschi, R. La Russa, G. Bertozzi, A. Maiese, G. Savioli, G. Volonnino and Y. Longhitano, "Cytokine Storm in COVID-19: Immunopathogenesis," *Medicina,* vol. 58, no. 144, pp. 1-14, 2020.

[25] C. A. Dinarello, "Historical insights into cytokines," *European Journal of Immunology,* vol. November, no. S1, pp. 34 – 45, 2007.

[26] B. Tuckey, "Fascial Counterstrain: A Methodological Advancement in Indirect Osteopathic Manipulation," *International Journal of Osteopathic Medicine,* vol. 58, pp. 1-11, December 2025.

[27] S. Barrientos, O. Stojadinovic, M. S. Golinko, H. Brem and M. Tomic-Canic, "Growth factors and cytokines in wound healing," *Wound Repair and Regeneration,* vol. 16, no. 5, pp. 585-720, 2008.

[28] S. Nirenjen, J. Narayanan, T. Tamilanban, V. Subramaniyan, V. Chitra, N. K. Fuloria, L. S. Wong, G. Ramachawolran, M. Sekar, G. Gupta, S. Fuloria, S. V. Chinni and S. Selvaraj, "Exploring the contribution of pro-inflammatory cytokines to impaired wound healing in diabetes," *Frontiers in Immunology,* vol. 14, no. 1216321, pp. 1-17, 2023.

[29] J. R. Zadro, M. O'Keeffe, S. Cheng and C. G. Maher, "What Interventions Do Physical Therapists Provide for Patients With Cardiorespiratory Conditions, Neurological Conditions, and Conditions Requiring Acute Hospital Care? A Systematic Review," *Physical Therapy,* vol. 100, no. 7, pp. 1180 – 1205, 2020.

[30] T. Field, "Why Am I Not Getting Better Even With Physical Therapy?," Form & Function Physical Therapy, 5 July 2022. [Online]. Available: https://www.formfunctionpt.com/why-am-i-not-getting-better-even-with-physical-therapy/.

[31] B. Patil-Takbhate, R. Takbhate, P. Khopkar-Kale and . S. Tripathy, "Marvin Minsky: The Visionary Behind the Confocal Microscope and the Father of Artificial Intelligence," *Cureus,* vol. 16, no. 9, pp. 1-5, 2024.

[32] P. C. Benias, R. G. Wells, B. Sackey-Aboagye, H. Klavan, R. Jason, D. Buonocore, M. Miranda, S. Kornacki, M. Wayne, D. L. Carr-Locke and N. D. Theise, "Structure and Distribution of an Unrecognized Interstitium in Human Tissues," *Scientific Reports,* vol. 8, pp. 1-8, 2018.

[33] M. Saraiva, P. Vieira and A. O'Garra, "Cytokines Focus – Biology and therapeutic potential of interleukin-10," *JEM – Journal of Experimental Medicine,* vol. 217, no. 1, pp. 1-19, 2020.

[34] W. P. Arend, M. Malyak, C. J. Guthridge and C. Gabay, "Interleukin-1 Receptor Antagonist: Role in Biology," *Annual Review of Immunology,* vol. 16, pp. 27-55, 1998.

[35] J. P. Shah, J. V. Danoff, M. J. Desai, S. Parikh, L. Y. Nakamura, T. M. Phillips and L. H. Gerber, "Biochemicals associated with pain and inflammation are elevated in sites near to and remote from active myofascial trigger points," *Archives of Physical Medicine and Rehabilitation,* vol. 89, no. January, pp. 16-23, 2008.

[36] L. Sherwood, "Chapter 2 – Cell Physiology," in *Human Physiology – From Cells to Systems – Ninth Edition,* Boston, MA, CENGAGE, 2021, p. 47.

[37] S. G. Waxman, "Basic Principles," in *Clinical Neuroanatomy, 29th Edition,* Mc Graw-Hill, 2020, pp. 7-8.

[38] K. Kusuonse and B. Tuckey, "Fascial Counterstrain: Convergence and Neurogenic Inflammation," The Jones Institute YouTube Channel, 14 November 2023. [Online]. Available: https://youtu.be/6U_vJXsxd34?si=kqsIWs3tegXZgYHP.

[39] W. D. Willis Jr, "Dorsal root potentials and dorsal root reflexes: a double-edged sword," *Experimental Brain Research,* vol. 124, no. 4, pp. 395-421, 1999.

[40] W.-R. Xie, H. Deng, H. Li, J. A. Strong, J.-M. Zhang and T. L. Bowen, "Robust Increase of Cutaneous Sensitivity, Cytokine Production and Sympathetic Sprouting in Rats with Localized Inflammatory Irritation of the Spinal Ganglia," *Neuroscience,* vol. 142, no. 3, pp. 809-822, 2006.

[41] J. Durnett Richardson and M. R. Vasko, "Cellular Mechanisms of Neurogenic Inflammation," *The Journal of Pharmacology and Experimental Therapeutics,* vol. 302, no. 3, pp. 839-845, 2002.

[42] Q.-q. Y. Yang and J.-w. Zhou, "Neuroinflammation in the central nervous system: Symphony of glial cells," *Glia,* vol. 67, no. 6, pp. 1017-1035, 2019.

[43] C. J. Woolf, "Central sensitization: Implications for the diagnosis and treatment of pain," *Pain,* vol. 152, no. 3, pp. 2-15, 2011.

[44] M. Echeverria-Villalobos, V. Tortorici, B. E. Brito, D. Ryskamp, A. Uribe and T. Weaver, "The role of neuroinflammation in the transition of acute to chronic pain and the opioid-induced hyperalgesia and tolerance," *Frontiers in Pharmacology,* vol. 14, 2023.

[45] M. Van der Hulst, M. M. Vollenbroek-Hutten, J. S. Rietman, L. Schaake, K. G. Groothuis-Oudshoorn and H. J. Hermens, "Back Muscle Activation Patterns in Chronic Low Back Pain During Walking: A "Guarding" Hypothesis," *Clinical Journal of Pain,* vol. 26, no. 1, pp. 30-37, 2010.

[46] A. Mukherjee and C. Ambar, "Spasticity mechanisms – for the clinician," *Frontiers in Neurology,* vol. 1, no. 149, pp. 1-10, 2010.

[47] S. H. Wilson, K. M. Hellman, D. James, A. C. Adler and A. Chandrakantan, "Mechanisms, Diagnosis, and Medical Management of Hyperalgesia: an Educational Review," *Current Anesthesiology Reports,* vol. 11, no. 10, pp. 1-17, 2021.

[48] V. J. Madden, G. J. Bedwell, P. C. Chikezie, A. S. C. Rice and P. R. Kamerman, "A systematic review of experimental methods to manipulate secondary hyperalgesia in humans: protocol," *Systematic Reviews,* vol. 8, no. 208, pp. 1-6, 2019.

[49] S. Chakraborty, M. J. Davis and M. Muthuchamy, "Emerging trends in the pathophysiology of lymphatic contractile function," *Seminars in Cell & Developmental Biology,* vol. 38, no. February, pp. 55-66, 2015.

[50] M. B. Aldrich and E. M. Sevick-Muraca, "Cytokines are systemic effectors of lymphatic function in acute inflammation," *Cytokine,* vol. 64, no. 1, pp. 362-369, 2013.

[51] T. W. Myers, "Fascia-Biomechanical Regulation," in *Anatomy Trains – Third Edition*, Churchill Livingstone Elsevier, 2014, p. 34.

[52] B. Hu and S. H. Phan, "Myofibroblasts," *Current Opinion on Rheumatology,* vol. 25, no. 1, pp. 71-77, 2013.

[53] L. Micallef, N. Vedrenne, F. Billet, B. Coulomb, I. A. Darby and A. Desmoulière, "The myofibroblast, multiple origins for major roles in normal and pathological tissue repair," *Fibrogenesis & Tissue Repair,* vol. 5, pp. 1-5, 2012.

[54] R. T. Kendall and C. A. Feghali-Bostwick, "Fibroblasts in fibrosis: novel roles and mediators," *Frontiers in Pharmacology,* vol. 5, pp. 1-13, 2014.

[55] O. S. University, "Anatomy & Physiology – 14.4 The Spinal Cord," Oregon State University, 2019. [Online]. Available: https://open.oregonstate.education/aandp/chapter/14-4-the-spinal-cord/.

[56] H.-J. Häbler, G. Wasner and W. Jänig, "Interaction of sympathetic vasoconstriction and antidromic vasodilatation in the control of skin blood flow," *Experimental Brain Research,* vol. 113, no. March, pp. 402-410, 1997.

[57] R. Larsson , Å. P. Öberg and S.-E. Larsson, "Changes of trapezius muscle blood flow and electromyography in chronic neck pain due to trapezius myalgia," *Pain,* vol. 79, no. 1, pp. 45-50, 1999.

[58] J. P. Fisher, . C. N. Young and . P. J. Fadel, "Central sympathetic overactivity: maladies and mechanisms," *Autonomic Neuroscience: basic & clinical,* Vols. 1-2, no. 148, pp. 5-15, 2009.

[59] V. Navadiya, "Structure of Lymphatic Channels & Physiology of Lymph flow | Role of Lymphatic System in Circulation," Nonstop Neuron – YouTube Channel, 31 January 2024. [Online]. Available: https://youtu.be/8Umj2u6A2fg?si=lZV8Zlb4oSDQqER5.

[60] R. Schleip, "Fascial plasticity – a new neurobiological explanation: Part 1," *Journal of Bodywork and Movement Therapies ,* vol. 7, no. 1, pp. 11-19, 2003.

[61] R. Schleip, "Fascial plasticity – a new neurobiological explanation Part 2," *Journal of Bodywork and Movement Therapies,* vol. 7, no. 2, pp. 104 – 116, 2003.

[62] S. Speakman, K. White, A. J. LaPorta, M. E. Payton, K. D. Gubler and R. J. Ryznar, "Cytokine fluctuation during acute stress is correlated to life trauma," *The Journal of Trauma and Acute Care Surgery,* vol. 95, no. 4, pp. 535-541, 2023.

[63] H. Christy, B. Tuckey, N. Miljacic, N. Polissar and M. Vythilingam, "Rapid Reduction in Posttraumatic Stress Disorder Symptom Severity after Three Fascial Counterstrain Manual Treatments: A Proof-of-Concept Study," *Military Medicine,* pp. 1-9, 26 August 2025.

[64] R. Spiller and K. Garsed, "Postinfectious Irritable Bowel Syndrome," *Gastroenterology,* vol. 136, no. 6, pp. 1979-1988, 2009.

[65] D. Zawieja, "Lymphatic Biology and the Microcirculation: Past, Present and Future," *Microcirculation,* vol. 12, no. 1, pp. 141-150, 2005.

[66] B. Ponikowska, M. Fudim, G. Iwanek, R. Zymliński and J. Biegus, "Harnessing the lymphatic system," *Heart Failure Reviews,* vol. 30, pp. 673-683, 2025.

[67] K. Kusunose and B. Tuckey, "FCS 101: Headaches and Head Injuries," The Jones Institute YouTube Channel, 10 June 2021. [Online]. Available: https://youtu.be/vAew4aq7FFI?si=ShNrPpMP27_sKG7_.

[68] T. W. Myers, "The Spiral Line," in *Anatomy Trains – Third Edition*, Churchill Livingstone Elsevier, 2014, p. 132.

[69] J. Meyer Berger, P. Singh, L. Khrimian, D. A. Morgan, S. Chowdhury, E. Arteaga-Solis, T. L. Horvath, A. I. Domingos, A. L. Marsland, V. K. Yadav, K. Rahmouni, X.-B. Gao and G. Karsenty, "Mediation of the Acute Stress Response by the Skeleton," *Cell Metabolism,* vol. 30, no. 5, pp. 890-902, 2019.

[70] C. Fede, C. Clair, C. Pirri, L. Petrelli, X. Zhao, Y. Sun, V. Macchi and C. Stecco, "The Human Superficial Fascia: A Narrative Review," *International Journal of Molecular Sciences,* vol. 26, no. 3, pp. 1-13, 2025.

[71] W. Mualem, J. Liu, A. Balu, K. Chesney and M. N. Nair, "Biomarkers related to hypertrophy of the ligamentum flavum: a systematic review of the literature," *Journal of Neurosurgery,* vol. 41, no. 1, pp. 33-45, 2024.

[72] C. Cunha, A. J. Silva, P. Pereira, R. Vaz, R. M. Gonçalves and M. A. Barbosa, "The inflammatory response in the regression of lumbar disc herniation," *Arthritis Research & Therapy,* vol. 251, no. 20, pp. 2-9, 2018.

[73] S. G. Waxman, "Anatomy of the Brain," in *Clinical Neuroanatomy, 29th Edition*, New Haven, CT, McGraw Hill, 2020, p. 156.

[74] J. M. Whedon and D. Glassey, "Cerebrospinal Fluid Stasis and its Clinical Significance," *Alternative Therapies in Health and Medicine,* vol. 15, no. 3, pp. 54-60, 2009.

[75] M. A. Neff, "Dorsal Vagal Shutdown: How to Identify a Shutdown," Neurodivergent Insights, [Online]. Available: https://neurodivergentinsights.com/dorsal-vagal-shutdown/. [Accessed 2025].

[76] S. W. Porges, "The vagal paradox: A polyvagal solution," *Comprehensive Psychoneuroendocrinology,* vol. 16, pp. 1-17, 2023.

[77] M. Avetisyan, E. Merrick Schill and R. O. Heuckeroth, "Building a second brain in the bowel," *The Journal of Clinical Investigation,* vol. 125, no. 3, pp. 899-907, 2015.

[78] K. Yamada, Y. Kubota, K. Kosaka, Y. Yamaji, S. Akita, H. Tokumoto, M. Kuroda and N. Mitsukawa, "Human Deep Subcutaneous Adipose Tissue Is Enriched for Inflammatory and Tissue Remodeling Pathways," *American Journal of Physiology – Cell Physiology,* pp. 1 – 45, 2025.

[79] D. LeBars and S. W. Cadden, "What is a Wide-Dynamic-Range Cell?," *Pain,* vol. 5, pp. 331-338, 2010.

[80] R. J. Meadows, E. D. Paskett, J. K. Bower, G. L. Kaye, S. Stanley and R. E. Harris, "Socio-demographic differences in the dietary inflammatory index from National Health and Nutrition Examination Survey 2005–2018: a comparison of multiple imputation versus complete case analysis," *Public Health Nutrition,* vol. 27, no. 1, pp. 1-11, 2024.

[81] I. o. H. Anatomy, "What Vaping Does to the Body," Institute of Human Anatomy, 9 July 2021. [Online]. Available: https://youtu.be/IaVaoja2Uk4?si=fRPA15Ngo3hgPOBJ.

[82] Harvard Health, "How sleep deprivation can cause inflammation," Harvard Health Publishing – Harvard Medical School, 29 April 2024. [Online]. Available: https://www.health.harvard.edu/healthbeat/how-sleep-deprivation-can-cause-inflammation.

[83] R. C. Burini , E. Anderson , J. L. Durstine and J. A. Carson, "Inflammation, physical activity, and chronic disease: An evolutionary perspective," *Sports Medicine and Health Science,* vol. 2, no. 1, pp. 1-6, 2020.

[84] Cleveland Clinic, "Poor Posture Hurts Your Health More Than You Realize: Tips for Fixing It," Cleveland Clinic – healthessentials, 6 August 2021. [Online]. Available: https://health.clevelandclinic.org/health-effects-of-poor-posture.

[85] S. Sikdar, R. Ortiz, T. Gebreab, L. H. Gerber and J. P. Shah, "Understanding the vascular environment of myofascial trigger points using ultrasonic imaging and computational modeling," in *2010 Annual International Conference of the IEEE Engineering in Medicine and Biology*, Buenos Aires, Argentina, 2010.

[86] M. M. Melin, J. C. Rasmussen, M. B. Aldrich, R. J. Karni, C. E. Fife and K. A. Eckert, "Additional evidence from a case report supports a novel hypothesis on the association between complex regional pain syndrome and lymphedema," *Frontiers in Pain Research,* vol. 6, pp. 1-9, 25 June 2025.

[87] A. Halili, "Temporal model for central sensitization: A hypothesis for mechanism and treatment using systemic manual therapy, a focused review," *MethodsX,* vol. 10, no. 101942, pp. 1-11, 2023.

[88] I. A. Sanchez, Artist, *Nociceptor Signal Pathway.* [Art]. Mar en Hoguera Media, LLC – Created in BioRender, 2025.

[89] I. A. Sanchez, Artist, *Types of Neurons.* [Art]. Mar en Hoguera Media, LLC – Created in BioRender, 2025.

[90] I. A. Sanchez, Artist, *Fascial Expressions.* [Art]. Mar en Hoguera Media, LLC – Created in BioRender, 2025.

[91] I. A. Sanchez, Artist, *Reflex Arcs Explanation.* [Art]. Mar en Hoguera Media, LLC – Created in BioRender, 2025.

[92] I. A. Sanchez, Artist, *Pain Signal Pathway.* [Art]. Mar en Hoguera Media, LLC – Created in BioRender, 2025.

[93] I. A. Sanchez, Artist, *Types of Cytokines.* [Art]. Mar en Hoguera Media, LLC – Created in BioRender, 2025.

[94] I. A. Sanchez, Artist, *The Interstitium.* [Art]. Mar en Hoguera Media, LLC – Created in BioRender, 2025.

[95] I. A. Sanchez, Artist, *Cytokines at the Interstitium.* [Art]. Mar en Hoguera Media, LLC – Created in BioRender, 2025.

[96] I. A. Sanchez, Artist, *Neural Convergence.* [Art]. Mar en Hoguera Media, LLC – Created in BioRender, 2025.

[97] I. A. Sanchez, Artist, *Cytokines at Dorsal Root Ganglia.* [Art]. Mar en Hoguera Media, LLC – Created in BioRender, 2025.

[98] I. A. Sanchez, Artist, *Cytokines Affecting Dorsal Root Ganglia.* [Art]. Mar en Hoguera Media, LLC – Created in BioRender, 2025.

[99] I. A. Sanchez, Artist, *Neurogenic and Retrograde Inflammation.* [Art]. Mar en Hoguera Media, LLC – Created in BioRender, 2025.

[100] I. A. Sanchez, Artist, *Neuroinflammation.* [Art]. Mar en Hoguera Media, LLC – Created in BioRender, 2025.

[101] I. A. Sanchez, Artist, *Tender Points.* [Art]. Mar en Hoguera Media, LLC – Created in BioRender, 2025.

[102] I. A. Sanchez, Artist, *Explanation of Neural Convergence and Motor Neurons.* [Art]. Mar en Hoguera Media, LLC – Created in BioRender, 2025.

[103] I. A. Sanchez, Artist, *Muscle Guarding Reflexes.* [Art]. Mar en Hoguera Media, LLC – Created in BioRender, 2025.

[104] I. A. Sanchez, Artist, *Cytokines and Fibroblasts.* [Art]. Mar en Hoguera Media, LLC – Created in BioRender, 2025.

[105] I. A. Sanchez, Artist, *Sympathetic Structures.* [Art]. Mar en Hoguera Media, LLC – Created in BioRender, 2025.

[106] I. A. Sanchez, Artist, *Direction of Ease.* [Art]. Mar en Hoguera Media, LLC – Created in BioRender, 2025.

[107] I. A. Sanchez, Artist, *FCS Mechanics.* [Art]. Mar en Hoguera Media, LLC – Created in BioRender, 2025.

[108] I. A. Sanchez, Artist, *Neural Convergence Analogy.* [Art]. Mar en Hoguera Media, LLC – Created in BioRender, 2025.

[109] I. A. Sanchez, Artist, *Inflammation Components.* [Art]. Mar en Hoguera Media, LLC – Created in BioRender, 2025.

ACKNOWLEDGMENTS

This enormous task came to fruition thanks to the love, dedication, and work of some amazing people to whom I would like to express my gratitude.

To my wife, Catherine—thank you for your unwavering support and patience in my journey to Counterstrain Mastery, but also in putting this book together. Your love and encouragement are foundational to my flourishing in this path. I love you with all my heart.

To Timothy Hodges—for opening my eyes to a new therapeutic dimension and for guiding me toward excellence. Our initial meeting changed the course of my career permanently and your mentorship has left a lasting mark on both my practice and my perspective.

To Brian Tuckey—for developing a therapeutic system that restores hope where it is often lost, and for showing us what is possible when curiosity and compassion converge. Your dedication is always inspirational.

And finally, to my clients—thank you for your trust and support through the years. Your courage and openness gave me the chance to grow, refine, and honor this craft.

WHO IS COACH IZZY

Israel "Coach Izzy" Sanchez is an author, pain therapist, and consulting strength coach who's passionate about helping you live a joyous, energized, and pain-free life. He started this path in the strength and conditioning field, where he earned recognition and exposure.

However, noticing how unexplainable injuries would manifest on the least likely of candidates made him realize there was a missing component on the physical-health spectrum and drove him into a quest for answers. Eventually, his own injuries opened his eyes to the limitations of conventional medicine and motivated him to research beyond the established. When his quest brought him to the world of Manual Therapy Medicine, he knew it would be part of his life.

Of all the forms of manual therapy modalities he pursued, Counterstrain became his choice because of its uncanny ability to resolve the most stubborn issues through highly precise, deep, but gentle techniques.

He has completed every Counterstrain course offered by the Jones institute and he's part of the first official graduating class of the Counterstrain Mastery Program—now the Counterstrain Academy—under the guidance of Timothy Hodges. Izzy also became part of the first official class of certified Fascial Counterstrain therapists in 2023, and also serves as Teaching Assistant (TA) during the regular Jones Institute classes.

Izzy values his privacy and when not at his busy practice or studying, he loves to read, grow veggies, strength-train, scuba dive, dance with his wife, or just unwind in nature.

www.ingramcontent.com/pod-product-compliance
Lightning Source LLC
LaVergne TN
LVHW070952210926
848482LV00002B/193
9780983566144